HEALTH CARE UNHINGED

The Making of an Advocate

LIZ HELMS

WITH ROSEMARY ROBERTS

PAGE PUBLISHING, INC.
New York, NY

First originally published by Page Publishing, Inc. 2016

ISBN 978-1-68289-731-7 (pbk)
ISBN 978-1-68289-732-4 (digital)

Printed in the United States of America

IN MEMORIAM

My inspiration for writing this book

My mother, Gertrude Davidson Urbach Taylor

Richard (Dick) Samuel and Linda Costigan Jr.

William H. Ware, DDS

Renee Paper, RN

DEDICATION

To all advocates and
To those advocates that are yet to come

A special dedication to all people that
suffer from TMJ. We have heard your voices.
Don't ever give up your fight for treatment.

To our TMJ Society of California Board,
thank *you* for your years of dedication

And lastly,
thank you to the members and steering committee,
CA Chronic Care Coalition

Many voices come together
when one voice stands up.
(Liz Helms, 2005)

CONTENTS

INTRODUCTION

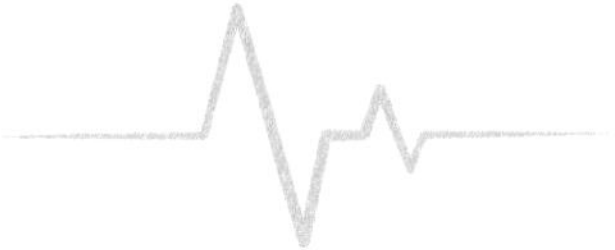

In the early 1990s, my life changed. I changed.

Due to an injury that forced a cascade of life-altering consequences, I discovered what true despair of the soul really feels like
and how within such a dark place lives a shadow part of our "selves"
that, if allowed to rise, can reveal a towering force of personal recovery and a true path of purpose.

As with any triumph of human kind, the journey is not one
taken alone and requires recognition of the collective good being
sought by all—the unity of both individual and collective passion for
a more just, accomplished, and thriving society.

I look at the world and the people in it differently now.

In my work as a health consumer advocate, I've been forced to
examine the motivations of others, those who hold powerful positions
of authority, as well as those who seemed content in a less just system
of status quo, never questioning, never seeking a higher authority in
themselves, and certainly, never asking, "What more could be done?"

And in doing so, I've discovered that everyone has within them
a hero, someone who can be motivated to play a role unique to themselves on behalf of their organization, company, or industry when
such a role reflects their personal story. If I've had an advantage at
times, it was because I was interested in knowing that story and gaining a better understanding of the individual themselves.

The road to advocacy is as much about listening, as it is about action.

I was fortunate to have had incredible teachers from whom I learned patience, as well as protocol, and whose invaluable experience allowed me to participate in and build coalitions of many, each bringing a knowledge and strength of their own to the table. The dedication and self-sacrifice I've witnessed is beyond words easily expressed.

My hope in writing this book is that my story will encourage you to go further when the road seems impossible to travel, stand taller when you feel beat down, and to seek out those who share your passion for change.

CHAPTER 1

Baby Health Care Advocate

It felt like someone grabbed a blowtorch and turned it on my jaw. The pain seared through the right side of my face and shot up to my ear, then wrapped around the entire side of my head. The excruciating pain was not from an assailant dressed in black, but something even more sinister: temporomandibular joint disorder (TMD), a dysfunction of the jaw joint. Headaches. Nausea. Vertigo. My life was a living hell.

And no doctor could help me.

Despite having health insurance from two different plans—my own and my husband's—neither one would cover treatment. Doctors said it was a dental problem. Dentists said it was a medical issue. I was stuck in a painful netherworld and thought I would go insane. I learned other patients suffering from this horrible disorder had already committed suicide, and I knew why.

I owned and managed a highly successful business called That's It Hair and Nail Salon, but I was barely able to drive to work. When I did, I often used the salon as the only health clinic I had. My head and jaw ached constantly. To ease my pain, I filled up one of the salon's ceramic shampoo bowls with ice. Slumped in a chair, I would lay my head inside the bowl trying to freeze away the pain. This was a favorite pastime now. Without proper health care, it was my one refuge.

From my skewed angle in the bowl, I saw someone enter the salon. It was Dick Costigan, a new customer. Dick and his wife, Linda, had come in to check out the salon and find a new hair designer. Their first impression of the salon owner, me, had to be bizarre. They both became clients of another stylist. It wasn't long before they began coming to me, and soon after, I knew why. Like many of my clients, they had become trusted friends.

"What are you doing?" he asked quizzically.

I rose slowly from the cold ceramic bowl, my frizzy hair wet from the melting ice. I could hardly talk, but I gave them a quick synopsis of what had happened. How I had my back adjusted by a local chiropractor and how the alignment had gone awry. How soon my neck felt like it had been torqued until it was so tight, I couldn't turn to the left or right, with tremendous pressure in my jaw. The same chiropractor adjusted me again, trying to fix what went wrong the first time, but he only made it worse.

I then visited my regular chiropractor who worked across town admitting I had made a very bad mistake and asked for his help. He adjusted me three separate times, and at each visit, he released more pressure from my jaw. During the second adjustment, I felt my jaw shift. Secretly, as my jaw healed—it "ankylosed," or fused.

One day, when I went to the grocery store, I started shaking uncontrollably and became dizzy. My blood pressure and heart rate rose, my pulse racing. I barely made it home and had to leave my groceries in the cart at the store.

Nobody could tell me why. I had no idea it related to my back adjustments, or my jaw.

The next few months were an absolute nightmare for me. After a flurry of doctors, neurologists, CAT scans, and MRIs, which indicated everything from a stroke to multiple sclerosis, I was absolutely convinced that my illness correlated to my jaw.

My primary care physician didn't believe me. This once-friendly neighborhood doctor had just been purchased by a large medical group and had both a new corporate boss and a different attitude about health care: "It will be a cold day in hell before your health plan covers a TMJ even if it was due to a jaw injury," he told me. I still feel a chill from those words today.

"You need to find another doctor," he added sternly. "It's the only chance you have." The best he could do was put me on Vicodin and muscle relaxants, which I swallowed like aspirin.

In my salon, I told this story of woe to Dick Costigan. I looked at him sadly with all the self-pity I could muster. "They treat animals better than this," I mumbled.

He was outraged. Outraged at the way I'd been treated. Outraged at this "new world" of mid-1990s health care, which foisted managed care on the masses. And he was outraged at my attitude.

"What's wrong with you?" he yelled at me. "Are you going to take this lying down, or are you going to fight for your rights?"

I looked at him blankly, my face throbbing with pain.

In the old days, I was a pushover. People walked all over me because I was too nice. I was a successful hairdresser with my own business who worked twelve hours a day, making other people look beautiful and happy. I was always the good girl, pleasing others. I thought I had no right to speak up. No right to complain. No right to happiness. And certainly, I had no right to good health.

During the 1990s, I lost my marriage, my health, and then my house—everything. I didn't think I had anything left to lose, but then something strange happened.

I lost my fear.

And I discovered something about myself I never imagined—I had power beyond belief. Power to stand up for myself. Power to demand the best health care possible. And power to take on a monolithic health care system that valued profits over people.

I've always thought it strange that suffering from so much physical pain could liberate me, but it did. And it would take me to the cutting edge of health care reform in California, which was eyed by many other states nationwide as a leader in patients' rights.

One of my comrades in this fight was Kassy Perry, who later said this about me: "Liz is fearless and has a remarkable moral compass. She will take on people and issues without regard for her personal wellbeing. She fights for what is right even if it harms her. She will go the extra mile to help a person in need regardless of whether she knows that person. Her sense of self is tied into who she can help and how she can right the world's wrongs."

How did I make the transformation from sacrificial lamb to tiger-ish health care protector? It wasn't easy. Although Dick and Linda Costigan, along with Kassy Perry, were instrumental in my future development as a health care advocate, so too was Dr. William Ware, DDS, in San Francisco who got me started by first saving my life.

I had gone to another doctor but never received authorization for the recommended surgical treatment I needed from my health plan. I received one denial after another, month after month. I was forced by my health plan to see in-network doctors, but none could really help me.

I knew Dr. Ware could, but he was out of my network.

My two health plans put more barriers to care in my way, and there were days I thought I wouldn't survive. But I had to. I had to keep working and pay my bills. I had responsibilities—a salon with a staff of fifteen.

Finally, I decided I had to see Dr. Ware no matter what. He operated on my right joint twenty years earlier, successfully. After Dr. Ware learned of my situation, he apologized for what I was going through. Realizing he might be able to help, he said, "No third party is going to tell me how to treat my patient. We are going to do surgery, and we'll work out the details later." We were a team. I had surgery a year and two months after sustaining my injury. My jaw nearly shut, my right jaw joint was unable to move and my left joint was beaten up so badly I had knocked a big hole through it. My mandible was hitting through the joint and up into my skull.

I quickly recovered from TMJ surgery and had to pay for it myself, which in 1994 was $25,000. There were plenty of other costs to bear too, including follow-up visits, medications, and physical therapy. I filed for bankruptcy, and in 1997, I sold my business to burst off in a new direction.

For that, I got help from two extraordinary friends.

My hair salon had always been more than just a salon to me. It was the social hub of my life. I designed and tinted hair while making an ever-expanding network of friends from my clients.

One of them was Layne Allred, a young, high-energy, six-foot three-inch family man with a crew cut who looked more like a former football player than the chief of staff for a powerful California assemblyman. As a customer at the salon, he saw me shrink from my typically high-energy, talkative self-working twelve hours a day to a pained, fatigued hairdresser barely showing up a handful of hours for the entire week.

"Not medically necessary?" shouted Layne, when I told him the story. He'd never heard of TMJ and asked me a million questions. Almost immediately, he started making informal calls from his legislative office on my behalf, applying "gentle pressure" to my health insurance plan. But they didn't budge.

"Then it became my passion because of the injustice of it all," Layne later said. He was the first to suggest creating a nonprofit association called The TMJ Society of California to represent patients with TMJ who couldn't fight their health plans single-handedly. Before us, there was simply no one who could fight for the rights of those suffering from this horrid condition. He'd been around government long enough to know that grassroots advocacy organization worked. Creating the TMJ Society was just the first successful fight in a series of battles we would wage together.

Layne signed on to my crusade and became the first musketeer.

The second musketeer was Pat Waltz, a tenacious trial attorney with an Irishman's passion for social justice. Completely fearless, today he represents common citizens abused by other attorneys. "If there's one thing I love, it's suing lawyers," he says gleefully. "Number one, it's a fair fight. They're really smart, and often times, they've done something really bad." Needless to say, Pat is not your typical attorney. He has an intense moral fiber that keeps him outside the legal mainstream. He works nearly solo in a vintage Victorian home, not a fancy downtown Sacramento office, and takes cases he cares about, not those that will net him the most cash.

Pat took the case against my health plan. I was determined to sue them to ensure they provided the coverage they promised to others in their benefits packages. Pat took a huge risk by representing me. He was not a personal injury attorney at all and took the case on a contingency basis when nobody else would. I was introduced to him by another attorney who declined because of a conflict of interest. When I asked him if he could recommend another attorney, he paused for a moment then broke out into a broad smile. "I know just the guy," he said.

Pat became musketeer number 2.

And I was the third musketeer.

The three of us, driven by principle rather than money, knew something horrible was happening not just to me, but to patients in California and nationwide. We simply weren't getting the health care we were promised. As I'd discover over the next few years, the problem was enormous and widespread. Health plans were promising coverage, then denying it. They listed insured drugs on their formularies, then secretly removed them. They pressured doctors to limit treatment. They demonized pharmaceutical companies. It was a frightening, corrupt game of health care *Monopoly*, and patients everywhere were losing.

As Pat and I drafted a lawsuit against my health insurance plan—which we knew would take years to settle—we worked hard to get the TMJ Society nonprofit status and a voice in the media.

"I can write up the paperwork," Layne told me, "but you are the voice." Layne also told me that the health plans hated negative media attention most of all, so that's what we were going to give them.

Layne completed the Articles of Incorporation to make The TMJ Society of California a 501(c)(3) nonprofit entity. Our first brainstorming session was around a kitchen table at a friend's home. Not a single one of us in attendance had health care experience. In fact, we had only one thing in common: all were clients of mine from the salon!

Later, at our first official meeting, we elected a board of directors. I was elected president...unanimously! (So exciting.) Layne Allred became our executive director, and my brilliant fighting attorney, Pat Waltz, was treasurer. Three others joined the board, Robert Becker, DDS; Brian Keropian, DDS; and Lou Gallia, MD, DMD. Dr. Ware remained my hero, and his office gave us our first check for $500.

We did great work in a very short time. Just one year later, we helped pass Assembly Bill 2994, known as the Jaw Joint Bill, which said that jaw joint surgery could no longer be discriminated against by the health plans. I testified before the California Senate Insurance subcommittee on behalf of the bill—the first time I'd ever done anything like that. Nervous, my heart pounding, I wanted to cry during my testimony (all I got to say was I support the bill). Afterwards, I felt exhilarated and realized one person could indeed change the system. Dick Costigan was right! I could make a difference.

The TMJ Society of California was becoming very well-known, and doctors began referring patients to us. Journalists were calling us for their stories.

And where did the phone for the high-class TMJ Society of California ring? At my station in the hair salon, of course! I didn't have regular office hours where I could devote my time solely to TMJ, so when the phone rang, I might be cutting, styling, or blow-drying hair. Once, I was mixing tint while I helped a caller get health care coverage. It was fun, exhilarating, challenging, demanding, and fulfilling. The TMJ Society was becoming a force for change in the state. We were following our plan to "educate and advocate": educate people about TMJ, then advocate for legislation to get patients the rights they deserved.

Overall, it was a crazy time in my life. My once-thriving salon business had dipped precipitously after eighteen months of illness, and I was slowly rebuilding my customer base. I had recuperated from surgery, was suing my health plan, and now was in bankruptcy. During it all, we were still trying to gain nonprofit status for the TMJ Society, which took a tremendous amount of time and effort.

But it was all worth it. Inside I was on fire, completely driven to change the way health care was delivered. I never had second thoughts about what I was doing. "Little old me" was making a difference.

And there were often immediate victories. One night, I was working late at the salon cleaning up when the phone rang. It was the TMJ hotline.

"TMJ Society of California," I answered.

"Hello," said a voice softly, mewling, full of pain. I recognized the sounds as those I'd made myself not long ago.

The woman told me how unbearable her life had become since suffering from TMD. She was in such pain every day that her life was unbearable…unlivable. Her health insurance plan wouldn't cover her; no doctor would treat her. She was suicidal.

I spent hours on the phone with her, describing treatment options and resources. By the end of the call, I convinced her that there was hope and that she had reason to live. She thanked me profusely and hung up. Although I never heard from her again, I'm convinced that I'd talked her out of suicide and that she is still alive today.

Probably the most exciting moment of my advocacy career—the one that kick-started my status in the advocacy community—was during a conference to discuss the future of managed care at Emory University. Emory is a prestigious college with a medical school located near downtown Atlanta, just a stone's throw from the U.S. Centers for Disease Control and Prevention, as well as the American Cancer Society.

The meeting was sponsored by Dick Costigan's employer. Dick had seen time and again managed care obstructing a patient's access to the care and the drugs that they needed. He thought it would be important for people at the conference to hear my story. I was clearly the poster child for the managed care nightmare.

Most of us don't remember how managed care was originally devised to provide patients a warm blanket of coverage "from cradle to grave." Instead, we hear the endless horror stories of severely ill patients like myself, unable to receive the treatment they needed.

As I packed my clothes for the conference, I was terrified…for a lot of reasons.

First, I'd hardly been out of California. In fact, I'd never once been east of Reno, Nevada. In many ways, I was a country girl, living in Sacramento when it was still almost completely rural and very much a cow town.

Secondly, high-powered legislators and government-relations experts would be attending the consortium. Not only wasn't I high-powered, but my only claim to expertise was intense suffering and a will to change an apathetic health care system.

In the car from the airport to my hotel in Atlanta, I remember a fellow with a Southern twang talking about the Internet and something called the "information superhighway." It was the mid-'90s, and I had no clue what he was talking about. I was a hairdresser and didn't even own a computer!

The night before the conference, there was an outdoor reception on the Emory campus, and I remember feeling very self-conscious. I was far from home. More important, I was terribly concerned about my hair! In the humid Atlanta air, my hair was far more frizzy than usual. In more than thirty years in the salon business, I'd rarely seen hair like mine, wild and untamed, typical of my Hungarian and Russian roots.

The weather was beautiful, and I enjoyed meeting thirty of the people who would attend the next day's meeting. They were all friendly and knowledgeable. I wasn't sure if I belonged with them, but it was good preparation for the next day's appearance. I had to put aside my insecurities (mixed with my anger at the health care system) and tell my story plain and true. I hoped they would listen.

I took my seat at a large conference table surrounded by an assemblage of legislators, health care executives, and government-relations experts.

My jaw was still sore as my surgery was just a few months ago. Although hardly anyone else notices my puffy jaw and swollen face, I do. When I look in the mirror, I can see that my jaw line is crooked, almost like a cartoon figure. In this setting, it made me all the more anxious.

As I look around the room, I'm somewhat intimidated by the prestigious gathering. Will I look stupid in front of all these people? "No, I won't," I tell myself. "I'm on a mission now. I have something they don't have—a story."

As I listened, the attendees spoke with intelligence and precision. Managed care was just starting to take hold in my home state of California, and the point of the conference was to identify growing trends and problems within this new system of health care delivery. But as I listened and watched, it was clear that there was something missing: a passion for common people and an understanding of what they actually needed.

To my left, another patient described her own horror story with managed care. She was a petite, fifty-year-old woman from the Midwest. Needing a new lung, her health care plan denied her coverage for a transplant. She was forced to organize a fundraiser to raise the $100,000 for the operation herself.

When it was my turn to speak, I was suddenly calm.

I tell them I'm a small business owner who was doing really well when I suffered a trauma to my right jaw joint, which fused the right TMJ. I talked about my eighteen-month nightmare of excruciating pain and frustration as two health plans denied my surgery, despite available coverage for TMJ. I described how almost ten doctors disagreed on a diagnosis, with some saying it was a dental problem and others claiming it was purely medical. I told these professional men and women dressed in their fine business attire that I literally begged my doctors and health plans to cover me because of the intense pain. Finally, I told them that after all the denials, a courageous oral surgeon finally agreed to perform the operation himself and accepted a payment plan that put me in severe debt. Most important, I told them about a health care system that is desperately broken and puts profits ahead of people.

As I finished, I was nearly shaking with anger. It's impossible for me to recount my agonizing tale without becoming incensed. And then, I heard something…people crying.

I heard Kleenex being pulled from pockets and purses. As I looked up at these powerful professionals, I could see a roomful of tears. I couldn't believe it. Every set of eyes was wet. After years of sickness and half-hearted care, months of physical torture and despair, of anger and apathy…these people really cared. They didn't see me as a piece of meat slapped onto a spreadsheet. I wasn't a number any longer, but a human being. They felt my pain. It was amazing.

Dr. Nancy Hall from Pfizer, the conference sponsor, rushes up to me afterward and said, "Oh my god, this is so horrible!" For someone like me who endured such horrible pain, it's an enormous relief to finally tell your story and know that people are really listening to you. Finally, I don't feel alone.

I heard more horror stories that day about managed care from people in government affairs, and I knew I was doing something that had to be done. I was working against a system that had to be changed.

Now I had a bigger purpose to my life. I loved being a hairdresser, but this was something more profound. I felt like a baby being born that day. I didn't yet know where I was going, but I knew I was on the right path. This little hairdresser from Sacramento, California, was on fire!

I was still on a high from the event and pumping with adrenaline when several people from the conference went to the Carter Presidential Center for dinner afterward. It was there that I got to know some of the others better. What I realized then is that these professionals weren't distant or unfeeling about the plight of common Americans: like most people in medicine, they just needed to see the faces behind the statistics.

Although I was not a fan of Jimmy Carter during his tenure as president, the Carter Presidential Center impressed and thrilled me. Outside the thirty-seven-acre complex was a stunning view of Atlanta's skyline. Inside, the facilities were luxurious and ornate, far beyond what I ever imagined. Live harp music played in the foyer.

We shared a buffet dinner together in the hall. I was still vibrating from the meeting and felt like I was floating through a tour of the center afterward. I remember most vividly an exhibition of past president's wives and the fashions they wore as our first ladies.

There was also something profound about the experience for me. Since I'd never been east of Nevada, I felt like a foreigner here, yet strangely at home. Perhaps it was walking through those halls filled with memorabilia of American history, or the sense of importance the center inspired in all its visitors. I knew that I too was going to make a difference.

When I flew home to California, I called everyone who had joined in my cause. Pat Waltz and Layne Allred were thrilled when I told them what had happened. When I called Dick Costigan, he'd already heard. "You were the star!" he crowed.

Dick's wife, Linda, told me to hang on for the coming ride. "You are going to be on top of the world," she told me. "Everybody's going to want to know about this. Seize the moment. Go with it because you won't be there forever."

Linda was right about almost everything.

I'm still here and loving every minute of it.

With the help of Dick and Linda Costigan and the three musketeers, we'd formed the TMJ Society of California. There was also a coalition forming on the horizon called Citizens for the Right to Know, which would ultimately force health plans to reveal *exactly* what they covered and what they didn't.

So far, all this effort was limited to California, but we knew the TMJ Society and the growing patients' rights coalition crossed all boundaries. We were determined to spread the word nationwide.

Square in our sights was the National Institutes of Health (NIH).

We knew the NIH set treatment protocols and standards that the rest of the medical community followed, but TMJ remained in the no-man's land of patient disorders: nobody wanted to touch it. For months and months, I researched TMJ and talked to Layne about my findings.

"Did you know that TMJ sufferers are 80 percent women?" I asked, looking at some papers.

"What?" he asked. "That doesn't make sense. Why is that?"

"Why is this affecting women more than men?" I continued, miffed.

Layne pondered the possibilities. "Do you think women are just more willing to be treated?" he asked. "Are men are too stubborn and prideful?"

I didn't know. At the time, there was still uncertainty over whether psychological issues played a role in TMJ. Certainly history had proven the great ease in which mental health (i.e., emotional issues) typically became a factor in most conditions relating to women's health, at least in the minds of the predominantly male professionals.

"Because we want to be definitive about whether it's a medical or dental condition," he asserted.

As I continued adding to my piles of research, I discovered that NIH was holding a conference on TMJ in 1996. It was called Management of Temporomandibular Disorders and was sponsored by the National Institute of Dental Research and NIH's Office of Medical Applications and Research.

"We have to attend," said Layne, with a wink. "It's NIH, and there are going to be a lot of doctors and dentists there with a focus on TMJ."

I wanted to tell my story, just like at Emory, but we weren't even sure if I'd get that chance. We knew there might be time at the end of the conference for public comments, so we took the risk.

In preparation, the three musketeers met and brainstormed a game plan. What was I going to talk about? Should we create a PowerPoint? Pat wanted to make sure the message was properly vetted because of my pending legal case. Whatever I said, it had to be succinct.

"You've got to speak at the end of the conference to make a big splash," Layne said. "You can't come up dry. You have to wake people up. Patients are in so much pain."

Together, we flew out to NIH in Bethesda, Maryland, expecting a sedate conference of highly intelligent and cooperative doctors and researchers. Perhaps 1,200 people attended the conference at the Natcher Conference Center, and upon arrival, we discovered that I was already on the list for public comments. Big relief!

The hall was enormous with a main floor and balcony. The first day, the three musketeers sat in the balcony to watch the festivities. We were shocked. What we saw at that conference was one of the worst spectacles of human behavior I'd ever seen. Attended by both academics and providers with expertise in TMJ, the conference was a sea of big brains with even bigger egos. I couldn't believe the things I saw and heard.

Instead of civil discussions about how to treat the disorder, we saw shouting matches between doctors! This was so strange to me because the doctors were supposedly there to share information and explore treatment options for TMJ. But they weren't doing that. All they did was try to make a point: their own. The bickering went on endlessly, back and forth.

"We thought this was going to be a meeting of the minds with everyone singing 'Kumbaya,'" recalls Layne. "We thought everybody would be working together. We were very startled to see this kind of fractious debate going on."

We thought the conference would explore the cause and cure for TMJ, but what we saw was little more than a fishbowl of clashing egos. High paid, respected doctors were bickering openly, spawning discontent, and behaving badly. They actively disagreed with one another and seemed to relish it. It got very emotional.

We couldn't believe it. Pat, Layne, and I looked at one another with the same thought, "Holy cow!"

At the end of that first day, the three of us went out to dinner, put our heads together, and decided to change tactics. The original plan was for me to tell my story. How I couldn't get access to the health care I needed. But we decided to try something much riskier. We had nothing to lose. Our mission was pure. We didn't come to town burdened with huge egos. All we cared about was giving patients hope to treat this horrible illness.

I had loosely outlined my original speech on a yellow legal pad. I threw it away and pulled out the big guns: my index cards. I was up half the night rewriting my speech.

The next day, there were still eight hundred people left in the audience. I was going to speak to them at the end of the day and felt a mixture of terror and exhilaration. This was a huge crowd, much bigger than Emory.

Six consumers had signed up to speak, and I was slated for the number 3 spot, but I knew what I had to say would be controversial.

I wanted to make sure it left a lasting impression with these doctors, so I let the other speakers all go ahead of me. I was determined to get the last word.

Before me, representatives from other TMJ consumer health groups in Massachusetts, Wisconsin, and around the country spoke. They showed slides of patients who suffered horribly from TMJ and writhed in agony. They told stories of friends who couldn't get access to treatment and committed suicide. Although they weren't angry at the people in the room, they were still very angry, with good reason.

Finally, it was my turn. As I stepped up to the podium, I looked out in the audience and located my fellow musketeers, strategically placed so I could find a friendly face on each level of the auditorium. Layne sat in the main floor directly in my eyesight. Pat sat in the balcony, off to one side.

In front of me was an alert system for speakers that looked just like a traffic light: green for go, yellow for one minute, and red for stop. I had five minutes.

My opening statement: I told them they were acting like spoiled brats.

"You know, you are all highly educated people in your field, most of you with advanced degrees," I said curtly. "You're scientists and researchers and health providers, and you supply all levels of care to regular people like me. But with your petty disagreements and squabbling, you are playing right into the hands of managed care! If you can't get along with each other and agree on treatment for TMJ, why in the world would the managed care health plans want to cover this painful disorder?"

All of a sudden, the room exploded with applause. It was the first time all weekend that it had happened.

"You're acting like children," I continued. "All of you have *got* to stop arguing and start working together because if you don't stop your appalling behavior, the people who matter the most—those suffering with TMJ—will never get coverage for this horrible disease."

Another round of applause.

I looked for Pat in the balcony. He wasn't in his seat anymore but was standing up waving his arms excitedly at me. I stifled a laugh.

The alert moved to yellow: one minute.

Next I told them about the TMJ Society of California and summarized my plight, giving them a glimpse of the hell on earth I lived for nearly two years, using all the research I'd gleaned over the past several years.

What I knew, even way back then, is never finish a speech on a downer because it provides no hope and no promise. "*All of us* must come together to find the solutions."

The alert flicked to red. The third and largest round of applause came last. It was thunderous.

I never made it off the stage. The NIH representative who organized the meeting raced up to me and gave me a huge "Thank you!" The president of the American Academy of Orofacial Pain was next and asked me to be their keynote speaker for their annual conference the following year! Behind him was a whole line of others waiting to talk to me. I felt like a best-selling author or rock star. Everyone wanted to say thank you and find out more about the TMJ Society of California.

Perhaps most exhilarating, some of the very same experts I'd read about in my research were now waiting in line to talk to me! I had gained credibility and earned their respect by conducting thorough research and using their language.

Sadly, although not surprisingly, representatives from the other patient groups barely said a word to me. I think they were jealous, or perhaps a little shocked by all the attention I got. I didn't care. We weren't there to win friends. We were there to change the world of health care, because if we didn't, TMJ would never be covered.

When Layne saw me afterward, he screamed "We did it! We pulled it off!" Pat's arms were sore from waving, but he too was bursting with excitement. We went out to lunch to celebrate…the three musketeers, swashbuckling our way through the health care system!

Afterward, Layne told me about his experience sitting in the audience, his ears wide open.

"There was whispering all around me," he said. "They were all saying, 'She's right…She's on the right track…Wow, she's convincing…There are problems on the medical and dental side and they can't figure it out…Wow, she's brave to do this…I can't believe any-one's ever suffered from TMJ that seriously…Is that really happening in our practice, that they're suffering, and we don't know where to send them?'"

In retrospect, I think my highest accomplishment was sending a positive message. So much of grassroots organizing is negative and adversarial. Although I was justifiably angry with the way I'd been treated, I've always made a point to work for positive change. "Let's work together to help patients" has always been my message. The bottom line is people. It will always be about them.

"That's always been Liz's gift to the movement," says Layne. "She is intelligent and passionate, will meet with anyone, travel any-where, and find commonalities, never too prideful or thinking her way is the only way."

Afterward, Layne and I decided to go to the Capitol about ten miles away. I'd never seen the halls of Congress, and I thought this would be a good time to go. I also needed to unwind. This had been such an emotional experience for me, and it took all my energy to give my five-minute presentation. Now I was on an adrenaline rush.

"She was just so surprised that she'd be accepted like that," Layne recalls. "She had come from a very dark, lonely place, saddled with all this debt and guilt and felt very insignificant and worthless…NIH was the zenith of her recovery."

In Washington, the Senate was in session, so Layne and I decided to go watch them rule the country. It took forever to make it past the endless security screens, but we finally walked into the Senate chamber and sat in the balcony.

Layne and I looked down on the senators below and were amazed at what we saw. Each one deferred politely, giving minutes to his colleagues. It was a shocking contrast to the conference. We came from discord and walked into the most polite arena possible.

I loved the feeling in that hall and eventually fell in love with Washington—the sense of importance, power, and prestige. At that moment, sitting in the Senate balcony, I knew this is where we needed to be. We were crusaders who were going to make a difference not just in the world of TMJ but the whole arena of health care. There was no question in my mind about it.

I realized we were also going to set the pace ahead of other patient groups. I knew this because none of the other groups had a positive approach. They were all so darn negative, always looking at the glass half-empty. Their slideshows about patients who committed suicide were horrifying, but they didn't offer solutions! Did they have an impact? Yes! Did they provide a solution? No! We needed to collaborate and have everyone move forward together, not count on scare tactics.

As we sat in the Senate hall, it finally hit me what I'd just done. My talk came back to me in a flash. Suddenly, I felt claustrophobic, and my knees got all shaky and wobbly. "Layne, I can't believe what I've just done. I've told a group of esteemed doctors at a national conference they were idiots!" He just laughed at me. But I was serious. I had to get out of there as quickly as possible before I fainted.

Outside in the bright Washington afternoon, I filled my head with fresh air. We eventually wound up on the back steps of the White House. As I looked back at the Rayburn Building, I thought of all the congressmen and their staff housed there.

"Someday, I'm going to testify here," I told Layne. "I don't know how or when, but I'm going to do it."

To Layne, it reminded him of the great Jimmy Stewart movie *Mr. Smith Goes to Washington*, in which a small town scout leader is named a junior senator and fights political corruption in the nation's capital.

"You start thinking about how blessed you are to live in a country where you can bust through these bureaucracies," reflects Layne. "You think that making change is something only the captains of power do, but Liz was able to come in and have a voice."

When I'm excited, I rarely sleep. All I do is work, work, and work some more. I work from the moment I wake until to the moment I go to bed late at night. My mind races with one idea after another, one project after another. Besides being president of the TMJ Society of California, I work with horses and helped found the Sweep Riders of the Sierras, a group of experienced equestrians that help with long distance competitive riding and are amateur ham radio operators. I also edit the newsletter for the TMJ Society and habitually take on more causes than I can comfortably handle.

As I got more involved with the TMJ Society, our legislative issues bisected with other patient groups. There was a huge need out there for consumers to stand up—together. Patients representing liver disease, Alzheimer's, asthma…these consumer groups and dozens of others needed to bond together to fight against the limitations of health insurance. Yes, I felt like the little hairdresser that could, but how far, exactly could we go? Turns out, a lot farther than we could have imagined at the time. And the ride? Nothing short of incredible.

CHAPTER 2

Anatomy of an Illness:
The Special Horror of TMD

Temporomandibular joint disorder, commonly called TMD or TMJ, involves inflammation and/or a degeneration of the jaw joint and the muscles associated with chewing. Common complaints range from mild clicking and popping in the joint to acute myofacial pain that worsens over time. Sounds simple enough, right? Not so fast.

The temporomandibular joint connects the mandible (the lower jaw) to the temporal bone, located at the side of the head directly in front of the ears. While these joints are flexible, allowing for movement up and down and side to side, muscles that attach and surround the joints control the jaw's position and movement. The rounded ends of the jaw, the condyles, slide easily within the joint socket and are aided by a soft disc, which acts as a shock absorber within the joint itself and keeps the movement smooth.

Injury to one or more of the jaw joint components can result in multiple disorders and symptoms, making individual diagnosis difficult.

Technically speaking, TMJ falls into three categories: myofacial pain (from mild discomfort to immense pain in the muscles that control the jaw, neck and shoulders—the most common form of TMJ), internal derangement (disc displacement, dislocation, or injury to the condyle), and degenerative joint disease (osteo-arthritis or rheumatoid arthritis within the jaw joint). As it's nearly impossible for one area of the joint to be affected without affecting another, patients often suffer from multiple conditions at the same time.

Few common conditions have endured as much myth, misery, and misunderstanding as TMJ. In recent years, some health organizations have begun to recognize the need for advanced myofacial specialties, such as the Kaiser Permanente, who now supports a full myofacial specialty department, and med schools are incorporating TMJ into their curriculum. Still, there is more, much more to be done.

The cause of TMJ remains elusive and treatments vary from professional to professional. Some dental practitioners believe in grinding down teeth to improve a patient's "bite" while others build up dental support with crowns or recommend an oral appliance. In the '70s, many dentists took an "all the above" approach, leaving a lifetime of dental chaos in their wake. Some recommend relaxation exercises or behavior modification early on, which may be beneficial to some, but futile if trauma has been severe. A patient's inability to open wide enough for daily brushing contributes to an overall decline in dental health, resulting in excessive cavities, exhaustive root canals and gum disease.

Even today, patients often struggle to receive the appropriate diagnosis and are subjected to multiple opinions and examinations as they travel the labyrinth of a struggling health care system, bouncing back and forth between dental and medical doctors desperately seeking relief.

TMJ is often referred to as the great impostor because symptoms vary from person to person and can mimic other, sometimes acute, illnesses. Mimicking a neurological disorder, for example, can delay receiving the proper care and, in some cases, cause adverse, life-threatening reactions in an otherwise healthy individual when drugs that alter brain chemicals are prescribed. This is to say nothing of the enormous expense involved when chasing multiple "ghosts in the night" symptoms, with or without insurance coverage.

All too often, TMJ mimics the symptoms of a wide array of conditions, including migraine and tension headaches, sinusitis, earaches, neck strain, fibromyalgia, chewing problems, lockjaw, neuritis, epilepsy, gastrointestinal complications, spinal problems, memory loss, and even vision problems due to nerve damage or impairment.

The relentless pain, often described as a 12 on a scale of 1 to 10, drives many patients to despair and depression. One's daily life, already disabled by the negative side effects of heavy pain meds and/or muscle relaxants, grows muddier with a pea soup of additional medications (including antidepressants) that may have little or no effect on the underlying condition. Unable to work, manage one's day-to-day responsibilities, or enjoy normal family activities, patients can become withdrawn socially, turning to self-medicating with drugs and/or alcohol.

Patients all too frequently endure endless doctor appointments, multiple rounds of medication changes, joint injections and other shot-in-the-dark therapies, emergency room visits for pain control, and an array of diagnostic exams (x-ray, MRI, etc.) that will prove inconclusive to the physician who's ill equipped to diagnosis TMJ.

Is it any wonder that for some, their world cascading out of control, the pain is ended with suicide?

While education and the diagnosis of TMJ has improved immensely over the last decade, dental and medical professionals continue to disagree on effective methods of treatment.

Even more confusing for patients can be determining why (or how) TMJ became a burdensome health issue in the first place.

In my case, trauma caused a rupture within the jaw joint. As it often happens, my many physicians tried to keep up with the acute (mimicking) symptoms I was experiencing and the worsening pain long before TMJ was finally correctly diagnosed. By then, the damage was done, and my options for repair were few, but that was only the beginning of my nightmare and journey.

Trauma doesn't necessarily mean impact, like taking a punch to the face. Many patients suffer from progressive TMD stemming from the "trauma" of having a tooth pulled, especially the more difficult wisdom teeth located closest to the joints themselves. If left untreated, often due to a lack of patient education or adequate dental/medical insurance, the condition worsens.

For others, it might be stress and/or anxiety that lead to grinding or clinching of the teeth, which over time weakens the joints and injures the muscles and tendons that hold the joints in place.

Teeth that don't line up properly (for a variety of reasons) can also cause an improper "bite"—an imbalance when you close—leading to added stress on one side or the other of the jaw as you chew. While popping or pain may appear one sided at first, ultimately, both sides are affected and require proper treatment.

TMD is the classic "which came first, the chicken or the egg?" syndrome, which can ensnare a patient in a battle over insurance. Is it a dental or medical condition? Did it start as a dental problem and advance to a medical issue, or was it the other way around? Did chronic headaches, trauma, or some other event create tension in the face and jaw that resulted in frequent clinching, or did clinching cause stress on the joints that resulted in chronic headaches? Treatment may be delayed as your insurance provider(s) battle it out.

The sometimes long and arduous road home from TMD begins at ground zero: self-help measures that encourage limited use of the joint and reduce spasms of the surrounding muscles and tendons.

The "do's" of self-help include the following: a soft-food diet that reduces chewing action, massage to increase circulation and reduce soreness, and good posture. Yoga and meditation are extremely helpful to the patient dealing with high levels of stress, often the cause of excessive clinching or grinding.

Other helpful tips include the following: avoiding crunchy and chewy foods, such as tough meats, nuts, carrots, large bites of food, high-impact exercise, and extended telephone use. When yawning, always support your jaw by placing your hand under your chin.

For many, the mild discomfort of TMD requires little more than home care comprised of heat and/or cold packs, prescription or over-the-counter anti-inflammatory drugs (ibuprofen or other anti-inflammatory medication) and relaxation techniques, such as bio-feedback, exercises or posture training recommended by an experienced physical therapist.

An oral appliance often referred to as a "splint" is used when creating space between the joint is necessary for healing. A splint is a clear, fabricated (made to fit) mouthpiece not unlike a mouth-guard worn in sports (but thinner) that snaps over the top or bottom teeth. In the closed position, a space is created within the joint to relieve spasms caused by tension and pressure.

Outside of acute trauma to the joint that can only be repaired surgically, joint surgery for TMJ is considered a last resort, recommended only when all other treatments fail to provide significant pain relief or improve jaw motion. In my case, surgery was the only option available.

For more information on TMJ—when to seek help and available treatments, as well as your rights as a TMJ patient—visit the TMJ Society of California's website, www.tmjsociety.org.

CHAPTER 3

Injured and Denied

After months of various specialists, multiple diagnostic tests and ER visits for pain, heart palpitations, and dizziness, the correlation between my 1993 chiropractic adjustment that had gone seriously wrong, and my acute symptoms finally came together. Ultimately, the frightening conditions I had been misdiagnosed as having, including epilepsy, were replaced with TMJ.

By now, one jaw joint was fused together as if cemented shut. The other was a cluster of dislocated and mangled bone sticking far beyond the socket into my skull. Surgical repair became the obvious and only answer.

After all I had been through, my instinct and desire was to seek help from the one person I trusted most, my prior oral surgeon, Dr. William Ware at UCSF who had previously performed surgery on my jaw joint in 1972. Yes, I needed Dr. Ware again.

Unfortunately, Dr. Ware was not an approved "in plan" provider on my insurance, so I would need to find another, competent oral surgeon.

Still, I was fortunate to be covered by two health care (HMO) plans: one, my primary policy from the salon and a second, as a covered dependent under my husband's work policy.

Because I was covered under two insurance plans (and because my previous jaw joint surgery was covered without hesitation), I assumed that surgical repair now would be covered with equal ease.

I assumed that my primary health plan would take the lead and that my secondary coverage through my husband would pick up any balance, minus of course, any copay on my part. My assumptions were also supported within both plan's explanation of benefits.

My primary plan listed TMJ as a covered condition, and although routine coverage for TMJ was excluded from my husband's policy, an exception was made when trauma (as a cause) was evident, as was my case.

In my mind, armed with great coverage and the correct diagnosis, the nightmare was soon to be over, and I was about to get the care I so desperately needed.

The sense that my long and painful ordeal was coming to an end, however, was dashed, as both policies quickly denied my surgery. Trauma, as a cause, was ignored or disputed. Both companies insisted that my condition was dental related, which was not only ridiculous, but also unfounded. My physician wrote letters of appeal to support diagnostic evidence of traumatic injury to my upper spine and the resulting jaw joint damage, but again, both plans denied my claim. Month after month, the cycle of appeal and denial continued despite a preponderance of evidence to support surgical intervention as the only course of treatment.

How was it, I wondered, that the expert opinions of medical specialists could be so easily ignored? Why was it that reasonable explanations supported by diagnostic images that the average five-year-old could read as clearly colored "outside the lines" weren't enough?

It was a process I would later become very familiar with in the world of HMOs, that of forcing patients to endure less costly and less effective, or ineffective treatments before approving what their medical professional stated was necessary in the first place.

Worse yet, it was a process in which nonmedical insurance personnel were making arbitrary medical decisions that often harmed patients by denying coverage altogether until patients and their medical providers simply gave up.

My husband's HMO finally agreed to pay for a new specialist to rule out other treatment options.

Knowing full well that one joint was fused solid and that traditional therapies would be useless, the specialist proceeded at ground zero and worked backward, forcing me to endure one painful trial after another for no other reason than to be able to demonstrate that surgery was indeed, the only option as a last resort.

An oral appliance (splint) was made—at great expense—despite not being able to open my jaw wide enough to wear it. After all, a fused jaw joint doesn't open simply because you "will" it to do so.

If you've ever experienced a mold taken of your teeth, you're familiar with having to open wide enough to have a large, metal dental troth full of pink goo inserted, and then holding your mouth open long enough for the goo to "set up" as a hardened mold. For me, it was a painfully impossible task for which the end result was known from the start. Once fabricated, the splint would do little but put added stress and pressure on an immovable object (my fused joint) and, in the process, increase my agony.

Next, in an attempt to reduce my pain level (not treat the cause, mind you), the specialist tried medicating (sedating) the "trigger points" of the muscles surrounding my joint with injections into the side of my face. As theories go, the medication was meant to relax the muscles at these trigger points of connection and, therefore, reduce pain.

While the shots were excruciatingly painful, the resulting sound alone sent shockwaves throughout the office as both the dentist and his assistant looked on with horror. Never before had they experienced a sound anything like it. My muscles and tendons, now bound tightly with tension and spasm for months, were brittle and hard like cold, thin plastic, and cracked under the pressure of the medication being drilled down beneath the skin. Needless to say, yet another useless, "alternative therapy" was tossed as ineffective, but only after I was forced to endure more suffering.

I was also sent for evaluation by a physical therapist that attempted to ease my pain through biofeedback exercises, massage therapy, and posture realignment.

All such treatments are common and very often successful therapies for the individual diagnosed with TMJ. However, in cases like mine where proven trauma and subsequent fusion of the joint had occurred, it was an exercise in delay, deny, and dispute that forced unnecessary and irresponsible torment and torture upon me. It had nothing to do with quality care and everything to do with cold and calculated cost containment.

I played by their rules and suffered the painful consequences, and still it was not enough. After all was said and done, they issued a final denial of my necessary surgery.

At this point, I wanted someone—anyone behind the iron curtain of authority—to have to look me in the eye and to have to witness firsthand my facial and jaw disfigurement, my features now twisted by battered bone and pain. And I wanted them to acknowledge, too, their role in my fractured spirit. I wanted them to have to acknowledge their role in my demise.

I went to the corporate office of the HMO and demanded to see the individual in charge of my case: the woman whose name appeared on my many denial letters.

Was I wrong to expect compassion? Wrong to expect that she couldn't deny her own eyes? Indeed, for a while, she expressed sympathy for my situation, she declined further consideration or discussion.

"What are these people made of?" I asked myself over and over.

Broken and now beaten emotionally, I had nowhere else to go. I returned to my surgical hero from the '70s at UCSF, Dr. Ware, in search of a miracle.

"I feel like a piece of meat tossed into the garbage," I told him. As a trained specialist, Dr. Ware was disheartened by the treatment I had received and the utter disregard for pain and suffering that our new health care system fostered. He was also furious that despite great advancements in the understanding and treatment of TMD, ignorance prevailed as a legitimate stakeholder.

At great financial risk, he agreed to perform my surgery and allow me to work out the financial details as a cash patient. How I was going to pay for his services, I didn't know, but somehow I would find a way.

What became clear to me over the ensuing months was that the distinction between a "medical" condition and a "dental" condition had been exaggerated and hijacked by California's managed care industry. It seemed like the HMOs had almost arbitrarily split up the tightly connected pieces of the human head—the teeth, jaw, skull, muscles—between two distinct medical professions and was using that split to deny not only my care, but also the care of countless other patients who suffered from TMJ with a known medical epicenter.

To my mind, this was discriminatory and all-too-convenient. Furthermore, managed care, which was still a relatively new medical finance and delivery model in the early 1990s, had been allowed to proliferate and mutate at will, unchecked by law or authority.

As I recovered from my surgery and attempted to rebuild my business…and my life, I began learning all I could about health care policy and the legislative process.

I remembered something Dick Costigan had said to me, "What's the purpose of insurance? If you're sick and it affects your ability to have a quality life, that's what insurance is for."

At the time, Dick had worked fifteen to twenty years within the pharmaceutical industry and was a regional manager for Pfizer. He had lots of knowledge and had been around lawsuits against his industry but also knew a thing or two about the insurance industry as well.

Dick likes to recall a John Grisham novel based on a true story about a young attorney whose sister is denied vital treatment for cancer—a treatment that the insurance company had provided its own executives, but not her. She dies and the brother sues and wins a $15-million judgment—a huge judgment at the time.

"This case," Dick explains, "brought several important practices of this particular insurance company out into the light of day, practices that, as it turned out, were common throughout the industry. As a matter of standard practice, the company denied all claims up front when first submitted—all claims, no matter the available coverage listed in the policy. Most policyholders would resubmit and appeal the decision, and those would be denied again as well. A dwindling percentage of those who received a second denial would again appeal and file a third time."

Dick understood what the insurance company was doing. Only those who pushed the hardest through at minimum three rounds of denials received the care they needed, which saved the insurance company a boatload of money. The rest accepted the unethical fate bestowed upon them by their insurance company and suffered because of it.

"The insurance company knew that if they were sued, they would ultimately only have to pay out what the surgery or treatment denied would have cost in the first place, so by issuing denial after denial, ultimately, there was no financial downside to the practice."

Of course, for those insured and denied, the downside was worsening conditions, unnecessary pain and agony, and for many, death.

In Dick's mind, I had no other alternative than to sue my insurance company…that or forever keep my face in a shampoo bowel.

I probed deep into the knowledge base of Dick and his wife, Linda, to learn how health plans saved money and how the legislative process worked. And I sought out those who were already in the trenches dealing with health industry stakeholders (policymakers, pharmaceutical and insurance companies, medical professionals) and patients alike, working for change within a system that seemed to have such little regard for best practices and positive outcomes.

I met with Joan Stevie of the Arthritis Foundation, North Eastern CA Chapter, who schooled me on the subtleties of health care coverage: which illnesses were covered by health insurance plans and which weren't and why. Joan was already a skilled warrior on behalf of patients with special needs who was influencing health care policy and exposing the black holes of arthritis care created by the HMO system.

Time and again, the same question rose from the depths of my soul: How did the world of health care and a profession devoted to helping people become so mired in a bottom line mentality?

The real question, however, was a more personal one: What was I willing to do to change it? Did I have it in me…whatever "it" was?

All I knew was that I had to move forward.

It was time to build a coalition of patient advocates, medical and dental experts, and legislative support to force HMOs into right action.

The TMJ Society of California was born—a nonprofit association that would assist TMJ patients unable to fight the system on their own, while also working to change the laws in California to mandate coverage of TMJ within the health plans themselves.

Just the thought of it was both exhilarating and daunting, but after all I had been through, it had to count for something. I had to count for something!

At the same time, as I became more knowledgeable about health plans, I began to understand that what happened to me was not only unethical but against the law. What I needed was an attorney bold enough to chart new territory…to become my legal warrior in a fight to make the HMOs do now what they should have done before, and more. And I wanted them to pay!

I wanted them to pay for the unnecessary pain and suffering I endured. I wanted them to pay for the financial losses I incurred to have the surgery I so desperately needed and to ensure that in the future, they would have to honor the benefits promised to patients within their policies.

Pat Waltz became that legal warrior, armed with a professional shield made of skill and integrity that repelled the threats of corporate maneuvering.

Together, Layne, Pat, and myself became more than just the three musketeers; we were the emerging architects of a trifecta of wins to come, the likes of which California and the shadowy world of HMOs hadn't seen coming.

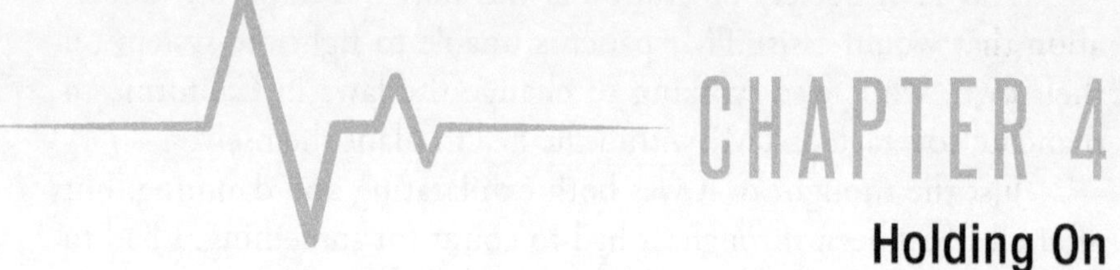

CHAPTER 4

Holding On

There's something about finding your inner voice…something about discovering a passion so strong that the very cells of your being begin to vibrate beyond anything you could have conceived. It's an amazing "high."

That is, until the natural skeptic within us begins to seep through, exposing old beliefs and self-limiting notions that caution us about our own perceived shortcomings. "Perhaps you're a tad out of your league…*just sayin'*," the voice in my head would whisper.

Was I out of my mind, or had I truly found my purpose? Did I dare really believe that I could be a worthy "voice," as Layne put it, and make a difference?

Sure, I was a business owner and, current struggles aside, a successful one. But was that, in and of itself, enough for me to build on?

Could I transcend the role of "victim" to become an educated advocate with enough audacity to challenge, and ultimately change, the landscape?

There were no idle hours in the day, no time in which my mind wasn't racing ahead of the sunrise considering strategies, partnerships, and making mental check lists for the TMJ Society, or nights without lingering concerns about the challenges ahead as Pat and I began to build my legal case against the HMOs.

Because my case would also set a precedent, I felt as if the weight and hopes of all who had been or might be discriminated against for

TMJ was on my shoulders. I knew that while my case would take years, it would essentially be just Pat and myself in that courtroom against a league of corporate attorneys sparing no cost or ploy to defeat us.

Sure, I had all the confidence in the world in my "David," but challenging the HMO Goliath seemed daunting, even on a good day. Despite my binders full of documentation, it was hard *not* to be stressed about the unknown.

Little in my world was recognizable, but at every turn, I was reminded of why I was in this. Somehow, the will to continue always revealed itself to me when I needed it the most.

My days were spent rebuilding my business at the salon to support myself and also pay the mounting debt from my surgery and post-operative medical care.

That's It Hair and Nail Design wasn't some small corner shop. In today's terms, it was a day spa ahead of its time featuring fifteen stylists, manicurists, and massage therapists. I was proud of what I had built, and it killed me to realize that my business had suffered such collateral damage.

During the most difficult period prior to my surgery, I hired a manager to keep things running in my absence and ensure that for clients and staff alike, the support and services that all had counted on would continue until I could come back.

As it turned out, apparently answering the phone had been simply too much to ask, let alone safeguarding an enterprise that I had worked years to build. Clients were lost, and business overall had declined considerably. Any chance of survival would demand a great deal of my time, energy, and resources, all of which were scarce.

Dick had wanted to get involved with changing the health plan system and originally thought a program more generically associated with consumer protection in its title was the way to go but soon changed his mind.

"Liz had two things going for her that was unique. She had a powerful story that encapsulated what was wrong with health care and the health plans and the ability to speak with people in both a passionate, but easy manner. For her to be successful, however, I warned that she had to tell *her* story…that no one could take it away from her, and above all, she simply needed to stick to the facts of her story. Don't try to expand it or deviate from it. Her story was enough and it was powerful. She listened and she triumphed, and she got stronger for it."

But now something else had change: the salon would have to double as the headquarters for the TMJ Society as well.

While a stylist is accustomed to juggling clients and working as if she has two sets of hands, I had taken things to a new level, adding secretary, media coordinator, and patient advocate/counselor to my job description, availing myself to fellow TMJ suffers in need of help and someone who could empathize with their pain and frustration. When the TMJ phone rang, hair dye and gloves be damned, I answered. When battered TMJ patients needed help with insurance or a "stick" to challenge their current insurance company on their behalf, I was there, battle gear ready.

Layne had filed for nonprofit (501C) status, and I continued to learn more about the underbelly of HMO plans, reaching out to other advocates, organizations, and associations that knew the system and understood the landscape politically.

The more I investigated the strategic and tragic mistreatment of patients and learned about health policy in general, the more I realized that almost every aspect of patient care was being compromised.

New words and phrases had entered the health care lexicon, especially for women.

Some were adopted as standard nomenclature by the industry itself. Others had become common slang that represented a widespread and sarcastic perspective of how the plans functioned.

"Drive-by delivery" and "drive-by mastectomy" were at the top of the charts, depicting the new cost-cutting advantage of discharging patients from the hospital as quickly as possible, preferably as soon as their anesthesia had worn off, regardless of whether or not additional monitoring or care would have afforded better patient outcomes.

Whereas today's new mothers routinely experience a visit from a breastfeeding counselor before discharge, mothers back then were lucky to remain in the hospital for eight to twelve hours post-delivery and be handed a pamphlet from the La Leche League on their way out the door.

Worse yet, the rate of cesarean sections being performed was skyrocketing. Patient advocates were concerned that the majority were unnecessary and performed simply to increase revenue for the physician, as an uneventful C-section garnished far more in payment than that of a normal vaginal delivery.

In the world of HMOs, physicians were forced to get creative if they hoped to recoup what they were losing in fee-for-service revenue. That physicians could plan their day and office hours around their surgical schedule was just icing on the cake. The surgical risks to mothers and babies, however, let alone the need for repeat C-sections down the road seem to factor little in the their medical decision-making.

While some conditions such as epilepsy were covered for office visits, often times, the medications necessary to treat the patient correctly were not. Some drug formularies covered medications considered to be less expensive but declined coverage for other newer and (deemed to be) more effective drugs. For many patients, failure to control their condition with the proper drug and dosage meant unnecessary and potentially harmful increases in seizure activity.

It was often necessary for a patient to try every drug on the list, regardless its lack of expected efficacy, before approval would be given for the drug their physician had advocated for in the first place. And even then, approval wasn't guaranteed. In the end, one could hardly argue that all those trial therapies saved money or enhanced patient care. Truth be told, patients often suffered needlessly.

As HMOs continued to replace standard group insurance policies statewide, consumers were forced to jump first and ask questions later...preferably never, placing individuals or family members with a pre-existing condition at risk.

Prior to a patient's enrollment, HMOs were not required to disclose what conditions and/or treatments were covered or excluded. Nor were they required to disclose what medications were on their formularies.

For my friend, Renee Paper, a registered nurse with extensive knowledge about the health care system, the inability to confirm coverage benefits prior to enrolling was not only frustrating—it was dangerous.

Renee suffers from Von Willenbrand's disease. During open enrollment through her employer, Renee searched through the documentation of the plans offered and made multiple attempts to ascertain whether coverage was provided for her hemophilia drugs. Despite her many inquiries, none of the HMO plans would confirm or deny coverage for her life-saving drugs…not because they didn't know, but because it wasn't required. In fact, they refused such information *unless* you were already a plan member.

Once you were enrolled (and had dropped your old insurance), they were more than happy to confirm coverage or break the bad news that you were simply SOL, "sorry."

For the average healthy consumer, doing one's due diligence to evaluate plans appropriately was difficult enough. For patients dealing with a chronic or life-threatening illness like Renee, they risked finding out later that coverage for their condition and/or special-needs drugs may not be covered at all.

For whose benefit was such a policy or, better said, lack of policy? How is "not knowing" what's covered before enrollment beneficial to the consumer? It's not. In Renee's case, and for many others, it was dangerous and also posed additional, unnecessary financial risk.

And more so, I wondered, who's allowing such nonsense? Who was protecting consumers?

These questions and more vexed me. Renee would later join me in fighting this, and many more insurance battles on behalf of health care consumers. Together, along with an organization called Citizens for the Right to Know, we changed the laws to reflect the protections needed.

Still, on a personal level, the challenges continued to collide.

My financial position made it impossible to avoid bankruptcy, and worse, my ex-husband and I were losing our farm property, which had been in his family for several generations. My heart was breaking.

We had exhausted everything after our split and now were looking to sell. Our realtor found us a buyer, and given that we were going to be carrying the paper, we trusted the realtor to do a thorough background check. It never happened.

Not only were the new owners later arrested for dealing drugs from the property, the place was ruined—our house and all, ultimately forcing us into foreclosure.

Like many who are faced with circumstances that leave no alternative, bankruptcy was another personal low for me. It was yet another situation in which I felt little control as time rolled by, my life in unsettled limbo…still.

After we had been in chapter 7 for some time, my attorney advised that it was time to file for chapter 13, which would allow a more favorable and permanent elimination of most of our debt. He cautioned, however, that the move involved a period of transition during which my assets would be at risk.

When the papers were ready, my attorney called to have me file them at the courthouse. At the time, my friend's horse trailer was hooked to my truck, and given that my vehicle was at risk of repossession if I parked and left it unattended, I circled the federal building for over thirty minutes while my friend ran inside and filed the documents for me.

I can look back on that day now with some humor—little ol' me dragging a horse trailer round and round a congested area of downtown Sacramento—but at the time, it represented my life somehow: me driving in circles, keeping one eye on the rearview mirror, while navigating the road up ahead. That I survived was a miracle.

But I did survive, in part because my name and that of the TMJ Society were gaining traction and attention. Medical and dental professionals were seeking us out, sending us their patients and getting involved. Our network of fellow advocates from the nonprofit sector and the politically connected was also expanding. Increased media exposure and requests for interviews was propelling our ability to educate the public and strengthen our messaging.

And I survived because I was no longer alone in the fight. I had my fellow musketeers and others at my side every step of the way, fueling my ability to navigate the system and grow into the purposeful advocate I desperately wanted to become.

Our "yellow brick road to Oz" may have been more like a hiker's trail in the Sierra's, full of cliffs and overgrown dead-ends, but we were together, growing stronger, more respected, and more effective with time.

We had shunned the naysayers, and by the end of our first year, I had testified before the California Senate Insurance Subcommittee and helped achieve our initial primary goal with the passage of Assembly Bill 2994, The Jaw Joint Bill—the first ever mandate anywhere to cover TMJ within all medical insurance policies sold in the state of California. Look, Dorothy! Why…it's the Emerald City, just there beyond the meadow! Can you see it?

CHAPTER 5

People Last: The Dollars and Sense of Modern Health Care

Inherently, people assume that if you're an advocate for something, you're naturally, 100% against something else.

In the case of health care, one who advocates on behalf of patient rights must naturally be against those stakeholders who are viewed by many as obstructionist in one form or another to the same; hospitals, pharmaceutical companies, doctors, and most assuredly, the insurance companies.

Nothing could be farther from the truth, for in reality, I have always recognized the legitimate role of each in furthering health care in the U.S., including the medical advancements that form the basis of our often envied care.

In fact, I could not have accomplished what's been possible without the coordinated and supported efforts of individuals who represent these stakeholders, nor could the changes necessary for our continued success in strengthening health care policy in California happen without them.

I'm neither a proponent of socialist values or anticapitalist. I'm a registered Republican, as well as a business owner who believes in the free market value of businesses large and small.

But, as with any "system," balance is required and all stakeholders must operate from a foundation of quality-driven responsibility for the consumers (patients) they profess to serve. When that balance is thwarted for…say, the sake of profits alone and to the exclusion of other vested parties, the system is placed in jeopardy and consumer confidence, not to mention the overall commitment to better patient outcomes is forsaken.

Health Maintenance Organizations (HMOs) were not new to the '80s but had instead languished in small numbers for over a decade, Kaiser Permanente being the oldest and most prominent membership model within the employer-based experience.

A for-profit business model, the ability of HMOs to break through the nonprofit legacy of fee-for-service insurance providers within the State of California, such as Blue Shield and Blue Cross, wasn't easy.

The '80s however presented a unique opportunity and pitch: as heath costs continued to rise, large group member-based HMO plans promised greater savings and increased continuity by coupling (in theory) preventive care alongside specialized care platforms for which primary care physicians functioned as health care managers. It was a one-price-pays-for-all, more-for-less proposition that quickly became like candy to the consumer baby.

Loved by employers for their competitive set premiums, HMOs were inviting to employees, who were quick to sign on to the promise of "complete care," agreeing to pay small copays for office visits, prescription drugs, and ancillary services, such as labs and x-rays.

In theory, having a primary care provider (PCP) managing the flow of care and referrals to specialists seemed logical and helpful. Instead of patients with multiple chronic medical conditions needing to coordinate the care of multiple, independent physicians, their PCP would provide the oversight…in theory.

For the HMO, the goal was reducing overall costs by ensuring coordinated care that would, among other things, decrease the likelihood of costly duplicates or unnecessary procedures, labs, and other tests and provide better management of prescription drug use. Further, because patients were required to obtain a referral for a specialist from their primary physician, the move also served to prevent multiple "doctor hopping," further reducing costs.

But soon, many consumers began to take advantage of the all-encompassing plans, seeking more frequent primary office visits, requesting additional and often unnecessary tests, and a greater number of new-to-market prescription drugs.

Initially, physicians were more than happy to comply but soon found they needed additional office support staff to manage the growing needs of documentation, including, but not limited to, referrals, consultations, and prior authorizations for treatment required by the HMO and more.

And the HMOs—as profit-driven entities with a fiduciary responsibility to stockholders first and sadly, foremost—began to see profits shrink.

Little by little, the world of HMO-controlled health care began to change, not by reining in excess or implementing known best practices that upheld quality outcomes, but by an industry that implemented disingenuous, slide-of-hand policies and procedures that were driven specifically and exclusively by profit motives—first with physicians, then hospitals, and finally, the pharmaceuticals.

First came capitation—a term applied to the maximum payment received by a contracted physician, hospital, or other care provider group on a per-patient basis by an HMO.

Capitation meant that a physician or physician group was paid a set monthly amount for each patient enrolled in a plan and under their care regardless if the patient was never seen during the month or seen multiple times. However, the cost of each lab, x-ray or additional office visit, etc., was deducted from the primary physician's (or physician group's) payment for that patient's care in a given month.

HMOs had effectively incentivized physicians to achieve more by providing less. They rewarded physicians who controlled the costs of patient care by keeping their patients healthy (or restricting access to services) and, in essence, penalized those who responded to a patient's medical needs (or request) for additional services.

Physicians were also given strict (capped) drug budgets, making it necessary to prescribe medication based upon cost savings instead of expected efficacy. Newer and more expensive drugs were less likely to be provided even when the benefits to the patient were clearly indicated.

Referred to as step therapy, patients would routinely receive prescriptions for the least expensive drug on an HMO drug formulary. If that drug was ineffective or caused severe side effects, the patient would receive another prescription for the next (step) drug up on the cost schedule. And so it would go until the patient had exhausted all the less-costly drugs. Only then, and often requiring delayed prior approval, would a patient receive the more appropriate and costly medication. The step process often took up to a year before a patient would receive the correct and/or clinically indicated prescription medication. Meanwhile, their conditions worsened and often became complicated by avoidable negative side effects and increased frustrations.

Soon physicians found it necessary to expand their patient load as a means of managing their financial risk; a larger overall patient load of less-needy patients would "in theory" insure against the risk of loss due to a higher level of care for one or more patients within the group. But as consumers increased their demand for additional medical care under the HMO system, in part because the system itself took longer to achieve appropriate results, providers of that care found it increasingly difficult to remain profitable.

In an effort to reduce normal operating expenses where possible and optimize every patient-dollar, cost sharing became the new business model of private physicians.

Small business owners—private, independent, single-physician practices—began merging. They began sharing staff, central offices and equipment, liabilities and more, and even sharing on-call duties, which were seen by most physicians as yet another demand on their time that they weren't paid extra for.

Instead of relieving much of the stress associated with private practice, physicians found they were afforded even less time and latitude with their patients. Because of pressure to see even more patients within measured and reduced time allotments, physicians were unable to thoroughly explain conditions and therapy options or to respond to patient questions.

Patients began to feel like cattle being prodded through an impersonal labyrinth of care stations without the trusted relationship they once experienced with their physician and his/her clinical support staff.

Increased patient loads also extended waiting periods to secure routine or emergent appointments, adding to patient frustration and delays in care.

Medical testing, the cost of which came directly out of a physician's monthly capitation share, forced physicians to steer patients away from expensive diagnostic exams, despite the need. Physicians who felt it necessary to order additional labs, x-rays, MRIs, and CAT scans, for example, saw a reduced reimbursement from the HMO. Once again, profit (even at the margins) began to dictate care, not best practices proven to generate better patient outcomes.

The squeeze was being felt by patients and physicians alike.

Capitation soon spread to the hospitals, where budgets became necessary for each and every department regardless of in-patient or out-patient services (ER, lab, radiology, ICU, telemetry, oncology, ortho, etc.). Each department became a separate entity of sorts, referred to as a stand-alone "silo," each independently needing to justify their services and associated billing.

While hospitals, like any other large business entity, had always been responsible for budgetary restraint, capitation by the HMOs forced each department to "squeeze" patient care costs further as a means to preserve independently mandated profit margins.

Maintaining independent budgets meant that spending more in one department because it would potentially benefit the patient and therefore, reduce costs overall, was no longer considered a standard of care achievement.

An additional diagnostic test or high-priced pharmaceutical, despite its benefit to the patient or ability to expedite treatment and healing, would often be forsaken as a means to preserve the individual department's cost-benefit ratio, as well as the overall hospitalization reimbursement. As each department sought to remain profitable independently, patient care was increasingly sacrificed as lives were pitted against revenue as the ultimate consideration.

As recently as a decade ago, the practice of withholding available treatment due to costs continued to produce tragic and unthinkable results in a country known for its advanced medical capabilities. The rising costs of new and improved pharmaceutical breakthroughs were the often cited as a factor in declining outcomes, as despite their availability, physician care teams often chose less beneficial, more affordable drugs.

My husband, Roger, runs a small test-only smog shop and employed a young man whose girlfriend remained in critical condition within ICU for an unknown disease. She languished for three months and was suffering from sepsis—a condition brought about when, due to one's body's response to infection, organs begin to fail in a cascading and deadly manner.

A new, yet costly drug, had entered the marketplace. It was expensive, yes, but clinical trials had proven it to be the only defense in grave cases of septic shock, such as this one, where death was all but certain without it.

I was familiar with the treatment and its known effectiveness from my work in pharmaceutical advocacy where patients were denied drugs due to costs. I pleaded relentlessly for her physician to order it without further delay. He declined, whether due to the drug's high cost or his lack of familiarity with it, I never learned.

The young woman died.

Capitation also applied to the payment received by a hospital when a patient was admitted...for any reason. They were paid the same dollar amount for the surgical patient in need of ten post-operative days, as the patient who was discharged after several days.

Hospitals soon began shaving days off the length of time patients remained hospitalized as a way to reduce costs and maintain higher revenue, often forcing early discharges on patients who were ill-equipped to manage their home care or needed extended inpatient care to reduce the possibility of readmittance due to complications, such as infection.

With the TMJ Society now in full swing and growing, and the passage of the Jaw Joint Bill behind us, capitation and all that denied a patient's rights and/or ability to receive reasonable continuity of care under managed care became our new battleground.

In hindsight, it wasn't difficult to see where, early on, patient behavior drove a great deal of the financial loss incurred by the HMOs, as patients abused and overused a system initially designed to limit personal financial liability while providing extended benefits of care.

However, the response of the managed care industry was nothing short of dehumanizing, forcing providers at all levels of health care to eat their own and ignore their Hippocratic Oath, all for the sake of profits and, in many cases, survival itself within their chosen profession.

HMOs began a systematic campaign of fear and coercion to keep their costs under control, destroying an environment that thrived on trust between doctors and their patients.

CHAPTER 6

Chief Executive Denialists: Inside the Mind of an HMO Executive

Being a pro-business, pro-capitalism, conservative businesswoman myself doesn't mean that I like (or condone) the behavior and ethics of all businessmen and women.

Indeed, when it came to the CEOs of managed care, the HMO executives operated within a self-regulated value system (or lack of it) that was impossible to grasp both personally as a patient, or as an advocate for health care consumers. When your own nature wouldn't allow you to purposefully carry out an action that could possibly, or worse, probably hurt someone, it's very difficult to understand the mindset of someone who could. Of all the realities I would face, the nature and operative mind of the managed care CEO was perhaps the most difficult.

Were they evil people? Certainly not. Were they heartless people? No. But the policies and actions they created and stood by to uphold the purpose and mission of their corporate entities *were* evil and *yes*, heartless. Nothing personal, mind you, just business. That's what I needed to come to grips with…*just business*. How was this possible? How does one separate 'who' they are deep down inside from 'what they do' in such a way?

Once a health care system of coverage provided by mostly non-profits where patient access and quality health outcomes were standardized factors, or at the very least, optimal goals, our health care delivery modus had suddenly become a private, for-profit industry driven by revenue.

Insurance providers were no longer foundations, but instead, corporate entities traded on the stock exchange for the prime benefit of shareholders, not patients. Patients were simply tools of the industry used to drive supply and demand of service providers, medical equipment, diagnostic procedures, and even prescription drugs, all of which were the basis of product (health care) transactions.

As CEOs, their responsibility and allegiance—and one could argue, their fiduciary duty—was to generate a profit, the more the better. Their jobs depended on their ability to protect the bottom line of the health plans and grow annual revenue for shareholders, nothing more. The measurement of success no longer applied to patient outcomes, but rather, what, or more specifically, how much needed to be provided while still spending less than what was collected in premiums. As the cost of health care rose, maintaining or growing revenue (profit) required spending less on actual care. For every dollar in premiums taken in, less and less revenue was spent on actual patient care.

Through artful, but confusing language regarding benefits, delaying or denying coverage on a case-by-case basis, or dropping coverage for certain drugs or procedures randomly without notice, a CEO could "manage" the ebb and flow of quarterly revenue and annual investor profits. These bright, successful individuals knew they were selling managed "snake oil" to an unsuspecting public who had yet to realize that their coverage was clouded by omitted details and unfair practices, such as what was covered when, and what was left off the policies altogether.

The results for patients were disastrous.

Health plan CEOs—with few exceptions—live in a world of boardrooms and executive suites, always with an eye toward one's personal, professional portfolio…where gains and losses are sketched in permanent ink that can further a career or demolish it overnight. Corporate America is fickle like that; *its business, ruthless business*, and the fact that a CEO is but human, has no place where bottom lines are concerned.

To survive in such a world also requires a dragon-sized ego, as one's success—defined as the value created for shareholders by their actions—also defines the "value" (monetary compensation) of the individual CEO. Ego also comes in the form of power: power over others within the industry and those who serve to carry out your will. Money plus power often creates the kind of dark wealth that serves the few on the backs of many, leaving little affordable room for costly compassion and healing purpose. The corporate ladder, being high and arduous, ensures that those below are vested in sacrificing whatever is asked of them, bearing the day-to-day fatigue that comes with being a subordinate tasked with doing the "dirty work" of the policy wonks in charge.

As CEOs throughout the state strategized and manipulated the health care system for corporate profits and industry dominance, they lost touch with those who were dependent upon reason and just deliberation by responsible people. They lost touch with patients whose lives were affected and indeed harmed due to the divided worlds of profits over care.

They became the guardians of policy for profit, unwilling to acknowledge the resulting harm and, shielded by the physical and theoretical walls of corporate structure, unaffected by the ravages of their actions.

While attending conferences regarding the many faucets of managed care, I would cringe at the words and notions I heard coming from the CEOs of health plans. They were clueless as to what was happening within their own hospitals and oblivious to the fractured care patients were receiving.

As innovations in medical technology and pharmacology advanced, delivering therapies with better outcomes and efficacy, the HMOs and their representative CEOs rejected such pathways citing high costs and calls of "experimentation" despite the potential of lives saved.

"How much is too much?" asked one CEO of me during a conference break. "How many new drugs do we need? How many new ways of doing things? When is enough, enough?"

My answer was short. "When we find a cure."

Inpatient, post-surgical hospital stays were being reduced by new techniques that were less invasive and allowed patients to recover at home quicker and safer. New medications were conquering illnesses that only a few short years ago were life sentences or reducing the side effects of more traditional drugs while at the same time proving more effective.

But to the HMO, and by extension, the CEOs, such advancements posed new problems. Rather than see the cost savings of reduced post-surgical hospital stays (and the related savings of fewer hospital-born infections), the CEOs saw a new surgical technique that was more expensive, never mind the benefit to patient outcomes. As for new drugs, what's a little nausea and vomiting or a few neurological seizures caused by older drugs if they saved money? Would they be forced to include the new drugs on their formulary just because they worked better, faster, and safer? What would that cost?

New procedures and treatments meant one thing and one thing only: the need for new, creative, and clever means by which to deny access to the same, be it through delays, disputes, or out and out denials as experimental.

Only when—*or if*—a CEO was misfortunate enough to fall prey to his own deeds through illness would he/she ever utter the notion of a lacking system. Only then would the words "dignity," "compassion," or "*medically indicated*" ever enter their vernacular. Only then would they understand that health care consumers are entitled to come first…that they paid to come first and have the right to expect more than delays, denials, and disputes.

Many Californians couldn't wait for each and every CEO to suffer a personal health crisis to become enlightened. They couldn't wait for a CEO to feel the despair of a parent whose child is suffering needlessly or the agony of an illness prolonged while someone behind the corporate walls of profitability delayed their care due to the endless process of appeals and preapprovals.

CEOs of managed care and health plans in general, along with their association(s), were quickly coming to understand that the TMJ Society (me) and my battle-ready band of fellow advocates from Citizens for the Right to Know and other organizations weren't going away quietly.

In fact, we weren't going away at all, but rather, we had won all of our legislative battles to date, had been getting a great deal of press, and were now showing up at every gathering of employers, benefit/policy conferences, and other health care associated gatherings we could find to discuss the need for greater transparency and coverage.

For their part, the CEOs tried to be cordial but rather came off a bit indignant of our presence, not to mention our message. Many wanted nothing to do with us at all. What right did we have to be within their midst and what expertise did we have in the area of managed care? At every turn, they tried to ignore us or at least downplay our presence and any contribution to the discussion at hand.

I can remember one conference in particular when I joined Joan Werblun, RN, chair of Citizens for the Right to Know at the time, for a gathering of large employers in which health plans were represented by a panel of CEOs in attendance. The purpose of the meeting was to lay out a variety of plans for large employers to choose from—those they would later offer to their employees during upcoming open enrollment. I was asked to speak on the panel and looked forward to taking questions from the employer audience.

When asked, the employers readily admitted that they selected plans on the basis of overall cost, not what coverage/benefits were included (or not) within the plans. In fact, they assumed most plans covered the same items and trusted that each would do right by their employees. They were, as most consumers were at the time, choosing coverage based on cost along with a song and a prayer!

Joan and I were determined to pose the questions that the employers didn't know to ask on their own, and in turn, enlighten them as to the holes in many of the proposed plans. We knew where the bodies were buried and wanted to force the CEOs to answer our questions…or at least try. In the process, the employers could make a more educated selection of which policies to offer their employees.

Our plan was effective but not exactly the means by which to make friends of the CEO types. Like irritating flies in the room, we took our rightful advocate place and drew ire with each additional question and/or explanation we provided.

Perhaps loathing is too strong a word, but anything less would be slighting the actual response of at least one CEO who found our position to be particularly unacceptable.

I was normally one to patiently stand my ground, while Joan was more of a "ready to rumble" personality who knew that to be there at all required the ability and willingness to engage on the battlefield, if need be. She knew that for the most part, we were in a "man's world," and if we blinked, our credibility and power to expose the plans for what they were and weren't would be lost. And she knew that if given the opportunity, the CEOs would come out swinging.

We managed to contain any heated exchanges until such a time that we were confronted out in the hallway by the CEO of the Association of Health Plans, the grand poo-bah of them all.

In the open-air lobby of the Hilton Arden Hotel in Sacramento, the exchange became quickly confrontational with fingers pointing and voices raised to the point they could be heard outside the hotel.

Joan was a diabetic nurse who was more than casually passionate about the needs of her patients. One of the many gauntlets she threw down that day involved what the HMOs termed "durable medical equipment"—typically walkers, wheelchairs, oxygen tents, or items that HMOs typically wouldn't cover, a fact that they all too commonly failed to disclose.

In the case of a diabetic, their medication (insulin) would be covered by most plans on their drug formularies, but not the needles they needed to inject themselves with, which fell under the carefully and purposefully misguided category of "durable medical equipment."

For patients who needed multiple injections per day and whose lives depended upon it, the cost of needles was often a barrier to getting the medication they needed. Joan would not retreat or be denied her opportunity to give voice to her patients, regardless the less-than-optimal location of the debate or public display that ensued out of her control. That she brought this item and more to light before the employers, forcing them for the first time ever to consider the plans carefully, outraged the CEO and his fellow plan executives.

Sure, I looked around at those who had stopped to gawk, measuring the shock on the faces of those nearest to me, and I'll admit I was a bit uncertain as to what, if anything, I should do. But in reality, I was rooting for her all the way, ever so proud. He was angry, yes, but only because we had exposed significant failures of the plans on offer.

It was not the first time we were challenged, nor would it be the last, but all of my colleagues and fellow advocates stuck together. We had each other's backs and stood united in our call for disclosure of plan coverage and patient rights, never backing down. We had earned our seat at the table, and California health care consumers were counting on us to use our position wisely. Still, it was rarely an easy undertaking.

As a patient who had been forced to fight the system and an advocate committed to ensuring that others didn't fall victim to the same, I was profoundly angered by the lack of accountability expressed by the corporate elites of health care whose claim to fame was profitability as a result of denying medically indicated and necessary care for patients.

No matter the views and concerns expressed regarding the system's failure to meet the needs of health care consumers, the CEOs often stood defiant with an uncanny ability to reject responsibility for the status quo and were equally unwilling to engage change, as either would require adjustment to their ever-protected bottom line.

When respect was due, I offered it by the bucket load. But I was quickly becoming educated to the art of respectful disagreement… and when necessary, respectful defiance. It serves me well, still today.

Health care is about people. When CEOs learn that and learn to lead their industry in a manner that affords a reasonable profit while also serving those whose premiums pay their salaries, our system of health care can thrive.

We can accomplish this and more. That's not optimism speaking. That's looking back at what was once considered impossible and recognizing how far we've already come.

CHAPTER 7

Demonizing Health Care:
Why You Hate the Pharmaceutical Industry

In the mid-'80s, America's love affair with the pharmaceutical industry began to change.

It's no coincidence that at the same time, we were in the midst of a changing health care delivery system that relied on controlling all aspects of care, including the prescription drugs your physician was able to recommend, all for the sake of profits.

A lot has changed since the 1800s, when in an effort to distinguish themselves from "snake oil" salesman, emerging manufacturers were called ethical pharmaceutical companies.

In the 1940s, Pfizer risked its financial future and reputation on a single drug—penicillin—leading to the glory years of the '60s and '70s when pharmaceuticals were considered the shining light of health care. They were viewed as smart, caring, and educated men and women in white lab coats. They were viewed as miracle workers, relentlessly committed to unlocking cellular, bacterial, and viral secrets in search of cures for some of modern day's most challenging diseases.

That was then, however. No pharmaceutical miracle could stall the tide of bad publicity to come, as the managed care industry began blaming the pharmaceutical industry for overpriced medications as a justification for limited formularies.

Before HMOs, patients and physicians enjoyed a great deal of autonomy, and choice of medications was considered a valued function of the doctor-patient relationship exclusively.

With an eye on revenue instead of patient outcomes, the new profit-driven HMOs began to control—dictate actually—every source of service/treatment a patient encountered as a means to control the total cost of care received.

With limitations already in place regarding a consumer's choice of physician and deep cuts to care and coverage during hospital stays, the HMOs stepped into the remaining frontier of cost controls, the world of pharmacology, limiting the drugs a physician could prescribe by creating lists of individually approved drugs, called formularies. Drugs not found on an HMOs formulary were not covered.

If a physician felt it necessary to prescribe a drug not found on the approved list, a lengthy process for prior approval was in place to address a patient's need. In most cases, patients were forced to first "try" the less expensive drugs despite their physician's recommendation and known failure rates.

Common, less costly drugs were fairly standard on most formularies. But newer, more advanced/improved versions of a medication, or those considered (and falsely described as) "designer" drugs with proven increased efficacy were not.

As medical discoveries and other advancements in health care came on the scene, such as controlling cholesterol as a means to reduce heart attacks, new drugs soon followed. However, despite their known effectiveness and life-saving capabilities, few were automatically added to a plan's formulary due to the higher cost of the new-to-market medications.

As generic drugs arrived, they also gained popularity on HMO formularies as "go-to-first" drugs due to their reduced cost, despite the fact that many generics didn't work as well for some patients over the preferred brand name product and caused additional, often debilitating side effects.

Formulary "tiers" were used to maximize profits. Tier one, for example, consisting of generic or older, less expensive drugs. A patient would need to "try" or exhaust the options available on tier one before a drug on tier two would be covered and so on.

Patients and the medical community at large began to rebel, causing a public relations nightmare for the HMOs. These corporate entities, however, were masters at creating alternative realities within the eyes of the public and began to push back.

First, they had to limit a physician's ability to offer trial samples of drugs not on the HMOs formulary—free samples that pharmaceutical representatives provided physicians to ensure a patient could tolerate a medication well before filling a prescription or to reduce out-of-pocket expense for those patients unable to pay for their medication.

Pharmaceutical companies were also coerced into pay-to-play deals. Those companies willing to pay—or offer special deals to a HMO—could see their drug listed on a plan's formulary. If they refused to pay what many considered nothing less than extortion, their drugs were blacklisted from the formularies.

Ultimately, by limiting doctors and the patients they served, the HMOs controlled all access to and distribution of newer and better pharmaceuticals and squeezed the industry for every dollar. By reducing demand through restrictions of certain drugs, the HMOs played a huge role in the costs of those drugs remaining high, but the public never heard that side of the story.

Further, while portraying themselves as the innocent victims just trying to help patients by controlling costs, they drove a negative campaign against manufacturers, convincing the public that drug companies and their research arms were the boogie men responsible for keeping new and improved medication just out of reach for most consumers. They warned that the costs of new and improved medications would drive premiums through the roof, something employers and independent policy holders were fearful of.

The health plan industry fostered a silent campaign of mistrust and embraced public relations myths regarding pricing, suggesting consumers were paying more for prescription drugs than in the past despite statistical data that could prove otherwise.

Today, most people continue to believe that pharmaceutical companies are nothing more than greedy mega-corporations who have driven prices to the point that many medications are out of reach for the poor and elderly or guilty of dumping lousy products on unsuspecting third-world countries as a means of recouping losses in the U.S.

But here's my experience.

While every industry has its share of unethical players, I worked with some incredible companies who placed a great deal of value *and money* on educating the public—helping people—which meant ensuring that ultimately, people received the proper medication for their condition.

A strange marriage? Perhaps, but pharmaceutical companies are often the best hope for many patient advocates, sponsoring health clinics and consortiums that provide further access and education to both consumers and the medical community.

Of great importance is their work with advocacy groups to educate themselves (and in turn, those they serve) in new technologies.

Specific disease groups (nonprofit organizations comprised of advocates who not only educate patients on conditions like asthma, diabetes, cancer, and seizure disorders, but also work with health plans and legislators to ensure proper access to quality care) vital to community outreach and are often able to accomplish incredible feats due to the education and tools provided by the industry.

Leading manufacturers have also designed patient-assistance programs, funded specifically to help patients receive the medication they need but could otherwise not afford.

In all, the pharmaceutical industry spends billions of dollars in research to make sure consumers get the best possible treatment, but we hate them because the health insurance plans have told us we should.

And what about those high costs for prescription drugs?

Certainly, the newest, most promising drugs are expensive, but what price do you put on your health…your possible cure? Would you pay a little more for the newest heart disease medicine developed with what we know today, or are you OK with a nonmedical bean counter at your insurance plan deciding that a few irregular runs of cardiac palpitations throughout the day, or the increased risk of a heart attack or stroke is worth it to save costs via yesterday's less effective drugs, or the future using DNA personalized medicine for the treatment of cancer and other diseases?

If a better, newer, and yes, more expensive drug could prevent or reduce your child's seizure activity, would you expect your health plan to cover it? In doing so, the cost savings overall could be found in fewer trips to the ER, not to mention reduce the additional health complications that could put your child in further, unnecessary danger.

Facts are facts: Out of every health care dollar, the amount of money spent today on prescription drugs is less than $0.12 compared to $0.07 in the 1980s. In three decades of countless discoveries and advancements, prescription drug costs have gone up only $0.03 for every health care dollar spent! When you consider the amazing advances in pharmacology and the benefits (lives saved) over those same three decades, I'd say we've gotten our money's worth and so have the health plans!

What has changed is the cost to research and develop new drugs and bring them to market.

In the 1990s, it cost $500 million to bring a new drug to market. Today, that price tag has soared to over $1 billion and an average of fifteen years of development. In only a few short years, that price is expected to climb to over $1 billion for a single drug!

With every endeavor, a drug manufacture puts a great deal on the line. Treatment for sepsis is a great example.

Sepsis, an often deadly condition caused a body's response to overwhelming infection in the blood stream, is on the rise with more than 750,000 new cases reported in the United States annually and growing. It's also the tenth leading cause of death. Far from just a disease associated with the aging, a simple trip to the dentist to have a wisdom tooth pulled can, in some people, lead to such an infection and cause a lethal cascade of organ failure for which even our toughest antibiotics can't control. Sadly in 2013, Layne lost his young sixteen year old son Parker to the horror of septic shock. I know others that survived but lost their limbs and must live with the effects of organ failure.

Now imagine that's your child in the ICU? Still hate the pharmaceutical company?

Drugs cure or control many of the diseases that have the potential to threaten your life or the life of someone you love, each one an expensive gamble to develop on the part of a pharmaceutical company. Keep that in mind the next time you request a prescription from your family doctor.

When I think of the number of Californians who have benefited from the advocacy work I've helped to advance—the laws we passed, the access to care we've afforded to many in need that was otherwise denied—I'm grateful for the support we received from all of our grantors.

There is no single bullet, no single area or entity of health care in which if we could change it, that would suddenly make access to care easier and/or more affordable.

Fixing our access to and delivery of care in California, indeed the nation, depends on all stakeholders working together and represents my most sincere goals as an advocate then and now.

CHAPTER 8

Hair, Hotlines, and Coalitions— The Right to Know

Grounded in our motto of "educate and advocate," the TMJ Society of California was making great strides. We had helped pass the Jaw Joint Bill in July of 1995, making denial of surgical treatment for jaw joints or upper/lower jaw bones illegal and discriminatory, constituting a misdemeanor, and our informal alliance with other advocacy organizations throughout the state continued to grow.

My name, and that of the TMJ Society, was turning up on everyone's list of who's who in local advocacy, garnishing invitations to discuss mutual concerns with other groups, and speaking engagements that could further our cause.

With every new venture, it was thrilling to see how far we'd come, and yet I had no idea just how much more was just around the corner.

If there were only one lesson I've learned that I could impress upon those who are passionate about a cause and looking for a way to move the ball forward, it's this: *jump*. And then jump forward again. They can be long or short jumps, but at some point, you have break contact with the ground and just go. And then make it a habit.

It's not important to know beforehand exactly the route you plan to take because the course will change in ways you can't possible conceive of, or control. Most often, they will change in much bigger ways than you could have imagined. Jump and the path will be shown to you.

If your passion is sincere and you simply take that first step, reach out to a local group or individual whose passions are aligned with your own. Believe me, the way will be revealed to you. It might be a chance meeting or speaking engagement or an invitation to collaborate with others down the road.

Meanwhile, don't quit your day job.

While attending to clients in the salon, I continued to take phone calls from patients in need and gave interviews in between cuts, shampoos, and color treatments. The media rolled out countless articles regarding my efforts with headlines bearing a common theme: "hair stylist becomes health care advocate."

But behind the scenes, while advancing my own agenda regarding TMJ, it was becoming abundantly clear that the voices of patients everywhere needed to be heard. What had happened to me (the seemingly routine policy of delay, deny, and dispute within managed health care) was happening to patients who struggled with every illness imaginable.

Regardless your medical condition, the roadmap to accessing the care you needed was often blocked, either through restricted access to procedures, medications, and delivery systems, or by a relentless void of information—one's ability to determine in a timely fashion what was covered and what was not.

Policies were fragmented and lacking details, and if you could manage to get someone from the HMO on the phone, they were simply unable or unwilling to help you. The sheer inability to comprehend a policy was astounding. The system simply didn't make sense and patients of all walks of life were suffering.

Dick Costigan and his wife, Linda, who had been with me from the beginning of my own ordeal, were also deeply concerned about access to information and care benefits in a more broad sense.

Dick suffered personally from two chronic medical conditions, and Linda was facing care issues relating to her parents, including her mother's cancer. A true visionary, Dick saw what we were able to do with the TMJ society and knew we could expand our goals if we united with others.

In December of 1997, Dick invited to me to an informal "brainstorming" meeting of sorts—a gathering of like-minded individuals who represented in some capacity, various organizations within the health care community.

While my efforts were more so concentrated on behalf of TMD patients and building the TMJ Society, Dick began to look into how the system worked for or against the average consumer.

Dick began to wonder, "If I wanted to enroll in a specific health plan, could I request to see the actual policy files for that plan by calling the insurance company or HMO? The answer from the insurance company was no…Well, at least not easily. I could, they suggested, call the Department of Corporations—if I was inquiring specifically about a HMO plan, which was regulated under the DOC—and arrange to go downtown to Sacramento to view what the DOC had been provided. I would need to make an appointment with a single individual who managed such viewings, and she was only available to the public for such one day a week. Of course, the average consumer not only wouldn't know whom to call for such information, they most likely wouldn't be able to afford the time or costs to take such action. Is someone from southern California gonna take a flight to Sacramento? Of course not."

Dick began to reach out to various relationships he had built over the years and individuals who, among others, were involved with the Diabetes and Arthritis Foundations and more.

He began to pool what was known about certain health plans, what was covered, and what wasn't, along with the costs involved with each plan. He made a chart: insurance plans down the left-hand column, basic benefits across the top, and the costs associated with the plans along the bottom.

When consumers were shown the chart and asked to evaluate which plan they would choose and why, most would admit premium costs were a key factor. However, Dick began to ask those with chronic diseases to consider additional factors, such as what was absent from coverage? What would those out-of-pocket costs, such as medication, potentially run, and in the end, were the lower premium policies a better buy or open-ended disaster for consumers? Further, how would they compare premiums to benefits if the plans weren't required to disclose coverage specifics?

"The more I learned, the more angry I got," Dick recalls.

"I learned, for instance, that it was standard for lots of health plans to hold their 'benefit seminars' for seniors at nighttime and always on the second floor or higher. Why? Because seniors had a more difficult time driving at night, and if they did manage to come, they were less able to climb the stairs to reach the seminar. The insurance company could say that they offered a benefit night to explain their coverage, but that seniors weren't all that interested in learning about the policy. Seniors would ultimately trust that what they needed would be provided…learning after the fact, that they had been duped, ripped-off, swindled and left holding the financial bag."

It was clear that a more broad coalition was needed to address the lack of health plan disclosure, resulting in Citizens for the Right to Know, but Dick knew that the TMJ Society needed to become fully functional in order for me to be effective and have legitimacy in representing RTK as a full member participant.

To that end, Dick was instrumental in ensuring that the TMJ Society had the funds it needed to achieve that end. Had it not been for Dick, my ability to move forward may never have taken root.

Dick's thoughts on our early history together regarding both TMJ and RTK are generous and gracious, to say the least. "By having such a strong demonstration story about the ills of the health plans, and the ability to tell her story effectively to consumers, state policy makers, and health plan stakeholders, Liz's involvement was essential early on and throughout the RTK's future and ultimate success."

Along with Dick, Joan Stevie of the Arthritis Foundation, Northeastern CA Chapter, and Joan Werblun, RN, of the American Diabetes Association, I began to explore how such a coalition might work.

While the day-to-day role of each individual/organization involved was typically to educate and advocate for patient access to care relating to specific diseases or on behalf of care providers, the confusion and difficulties surrounding covered benefits within the HMO plans themselves was something that collectively, all struggled with and had a stake in addressing. Joining forces to form a singular, more powerful voice was brilliant, exciting, and inspiring.

Beyond the TMJ Society, there was potential to become part of a coalition that would actually be taking on the HMOs in a much bigger way. Once again, my mind raced with ideas born of both fear (can I do this?) and excitement (I'm doing this!), only this time, the latter outweighed the former. I was stronger. I had grown. I was ready for more.

I was an advocate, as well as someone who knew firsthand the level of frustration and unnecessary pain that others were being forced to endure, and it was clear that there was a role I could play in this emerging coalition of organizations, which would later become known as Citizens for the Right to Know—an important umbrella organization that brought a host of statewide health care advocates together on behalf of patient rights.

RTK, as we often referred to it, introduced me to an even wider community within health care (the power players, and yes, the obstructionists) and afforded me even greater credibility within the advocacy arena.

Within the group, I represented the TMJ Society as a member organization and used my own voice as a patient who could speak directly and personally about the issues affecting all patients. It was my story but also the story of many.

Joan Stevie, who proved to be the grounding force of RTK's mission over the years, always ensuring that we kept to our foundation of purpose, recalls the early years as confusing for patients and advocates alike. "We were all struggling to understand the various plans and policies. It was impossible to guide our patients in the right direction when it came to selecting a plan because, as advocates and professionals who had a great capacity to grasp the language, even we couldn't determine what was covered and what wasn't. How could we expect the average consumer to understand them, let alone, choose a policy wisely based upon the best available coverage for their families?"

Joan, describing the problems as "global in nature," would often testify to the manner in which the lack of basic information afforded by the health plans (explaining covered benefits or disclosing what wasn't covered) presented a barrier that was universal to all consumers, regardless their need or chronic health condition.

Eventually comprising more than eighty large and small patient and provider advocacy organizations, including the Alzheimer's Association, the American Liver Foundation, the California Medical Association, and the California Dental Association, the collective mission of the group and our demand of the HMO industry was united in cause: disclosure.

When asked to describe the goal of Citizens for the Right to Know, it was pretty simple: "We want to shine a bright light on managed care and force the industry to spell out what California consumers can expect from their health plan…in plain English."

We wanted laws on the books that would force the health plans to clearly indicate exactly what they covered and what they didn't.

We wanted health consumers to be able to compare plans and make informed decisions about which plan met the needs of their family *before* joining a HMO or spending $1 in premiums.

We wanted laws that stated an HMO must put in writing which procedures and treatments were covered and which weren't, which drugs were on their formularies, including their policy for access to off-formulary drugs, and any appeal or prior authorization process required if necessary.

Citizens for the Right to Know became very active in the community, educating consumers to the pitfalls of current plans, and how to overcome them. We were building an army of consumers, arming them with information and asking them to join our cause.

We took our message and our campaign for change public and racked up success after success to the dismay of the HMOs.

We attended meetings with senior citizens and others and would help them ask the right questions of health plans:

- Can I see the doctor of my choice?

- Will the HMO cover the medicines I need *without* restrictions?
- Does the HMO place financial pressure on my doctor and limit my access to care?
- What happens if I travel out of state? Do you have coverage?
- How do you know if there's a cap on my prescription drugs?
- Is there a lifetime cap on my medical expenses?

Personally, I had traveled so far, and it was a powerful feeling knowing that I was a part of something huge—part of something "right" in health care and helping others to feel empowered as well. But still, I was a very angry activist, and I wasn't alone.

Joan Werblun, RN, founder of the American Diabetes Association, Sacramento, scoffed and howled at the absurdity of what patients with diabetes were going through. "If you have diabetes, they'll give you the insulin you need, but not the injector—the needles!" She was absolutely furious at the insanity of the health plans and their coverage. Couldn't the HMOs see and understand what they were doing to people?

Did we need crayons and paper to draw them a picture?

No, the HMOs knew exactly what they were doing and had little, if any, regard for the pain and suffering that resulted from their actions, always guided instead by the almighty bottom line and the dollars associated with it.

What we needed was legislation and an authoritative body with spine—the means by which California could lay down the ground rules for managed care in our state and the power to enforce those rules.

RTK rapidly grew in both strength and support, winning several important battles during this period.

We met with the Department of Corporations (DOC) who had jurisdiction over HMOs to help establish the new Department of Managed Health Care, which would oversee and regulate health plans. This was a huge victory and vital to our goals!

Regulation of the HMOs fell to the DOC beginning in the mid-'70s after a less proactive state regulator with limited authority had failed, leaving fraud and abuse spiraling out of control.

The DOC was better suited because they (HMOs) were not insurance companies, but private corporations—businesses.

As corporations, HMOs needed to be governed by a state agency that understood corporate entities and also had the staffing, legal professionals, prowess, and wherewithal to enforce the rules that govern corporations.

The DOC was the only state agency more experienced with regulating businesses that also had the resources and legal authority to clean up the industry. Their legal teams could go to court without needing assistance from (or the blessing of) the attorney general's office.

Still, managed care was an emerging yet transforming system of health care delivery, and as the saying goes, Rome wasn't built in a day.

Due to its "potential" for enormous costs savings, new regulations were given thoughtful consideration as to not encumber the process more than it need be. Still, many of the laws already on the books were not being followed, and more were needed.

It took time and pressure (political and public), and the blood, sweat, and tears of the grass roots movement to educate the agency as to the needs of health care consumers and force the HMO plans to change their ways.

Several years earlier, I had met a wonderful attorney within the DOC by the name of Warren Barnes. Warren understood that people are not commodities to be traded or stock options to be bundled and sold for profit or, worse, left to fend for themselves or die.

Lives were at stake, and once engaged, Warren and the DOC responded, creating the Department of Managed Care.

Today, the Department of Managed Care of California remains the most aggressive state agency overseeing HMOs in the country, supporting the strongest patient rights laws in our nation.

According to Warren, California has been able to maintain costs more effectively than any other states in part due to our laws that require (where applicable) preventative care.

"Medicare could have saved a great deal of money if the federal government had passed nationally mandated preventative care measures long ago. Preventative care fosters better management of patient health issues, including chronic medical conditions, and relies heavily on known best practices. But unless it's mandated by the federal government—as Medicare is a federal program—states won't, on their own, pay for preventative care upfront, despite the overwhelming cost savings on the back end."

Warren has been one of my most trusted, vital allies over the years, continuing today to serve with me as a member of the California Chronic Care Coalition (more on that later), helping to further our goals for better access to quality care, better health outcomes, and a more just system of medical care delivery.

We also helped to establish the statewide Office of the Patient Advocate, the first such advocacy office in the country. The office, which is part of DHMC, is responsible for addressing consumer concerns and complaints and helping bring action against those who abused their authority. Patients who feel victimized by their HMO no longer need to become experts in health policy. They have an advocate who can cut through the red tape on their behalf, something else most states don't provide for their resident consumers.

The HMOs continued to exercise their power whenever and wherever they could, but we had momentum and weren't about to turn back.

We fought "gag orders" preventing doctors from providing complete health care information to patients. While the health plans said they weren't engaged in such activity, we were able to prove they were literally preventing doctors from speaking freely and informing patients of all the treatment options available to them. If a patient didn't know about a new procedure or medication—one that might also cost more—the HMO could avoid paying for it.

Drugs and the plan formularies also continued to be of great concern for RTK. Through countless stories we were hearing from patients, we determined that the health plans were dropping drugs off their formularies without notice. Subsequently, RTK requested that the Department of Corporations investigate. The DOC confirmed our claims and issued a "cease and desist" order to the health plans during a hot and ugly press conference.

Did I say that momentum was on our side? Well, that and the full force of the state in some cases, and we weren't nearly done.

The Government Accountability Office (GAO) in Washington took note of what we were doing in California and launched its own nationwide investigation into drug formularies on behalf of plans that fell under federal regulations, such as Medicare.

At their request, I lived my dream and testified before the Congress on the matter. Yes, indeed…I had arrived in the big leagues!

Ultimately, the GAO report substantiated our findings and found that four categories of drugs were being discriminated against: cardiovascular, anti-depression, cholesterol and gastrointestinal (stomach).

Where health plan drug formularies were concerned, there was no place left to hide!

Next, RTK was joined by several other organizations and turned up the heat by taking out full-page ads in newspapers, including *The Los Angeles Times*, featuring me with the headline, "When It Comes to Your HMO…What You Don't Know Might Hurt You." The ads were part of the "HMO Oh-No!" campaign and went on to read, "The choice of a health plan is too serious of a decision to make without knowing the facts—the wrong choice can be deadly."

The more California consumers began to hear about managed care and learned of the horror stories that were becoming commonplace, the more they began to ask questions. Furthermore, they no longer remained silently willing to accept whatever ridiculous answer their plan administrator told them. If it smelled fishy, they went looking for answers from RTK, the Patient Advocate's office, or the Department of Managed Care.

Finally, consumers had the resources they needed to at least get answers and hopefully the care they were seeking.

Citizens for the Right To Know had opened up a whole new area of privilege for me—the ability to raise my voice again and again for the rights of patients. But for all our success, the road to protecting patients by means of proper disclosure within health plans and access to open, realistic, and appropriate information from one's physician wasn't paved with yellow bricks or folksy song. It was hard won within a plethora of competing and often opposing interests, each jockeying to maintain positioning while the world of health care transformed around them.

Dick remained what he likes to call "an unofficial member" of RTK and for a very good reason. He was doing something no one from his industry had done before, which was to step into consumer rights and speak truth to power within an industry that had a great deal to lose.

Had one of the health plans found out that Dick was behind some of the internal intelligence of RTK. "My company would have fired me on the spot," Dick admits, "rather than risk the insurance plans removing all of our products from their formulary until and unless they got rid of me."

Still, it's amazing to look back at what he was able to accomplish. While still operating under the radar of his employer, Dick was able to help develop "best practices" around the world, and with what he learned while helping to build out the TMJ Society and RTK, he was able to help other organizations around the country build similar consumer rights organizations within their individual states.

Using my story and what we had accomplished together, Dick would enlighten other voluntary health associations, all with members who suffered acute and chronic health conditions, about our success in California.

As it often happened, specific gatherings (conferences involving such groups) would include state, local, and/or federal government health officials who, either by ignorance or industry influence, preferred not to rock the boat and instead, keep the status quo. Dick felt it his responsibility—and opportunity—to set the record straight… all part of his next-step goals, where to take his message from here.

One of my favorite stories involving Dick's passion and willingness to stand up and be heard on behalf of consumers involved one such gathering in Seattle, Washington.

The story reflects what was often the case; the wrong people were involved in making decisions about the needs of patients without having a clue about what these decisions actually involved, or worse, their consequences.

I remember a very young woman from the White House speaking, Dick recounts, telling the groups represented how good and healthy they all looked... so good and healthy in fact that they wouldn't cost much money—a good thing! Recognizing her life experience as limited, and considering that these people all represented patients who suffered greatly, I couldn't take it and had to speak up.

"Excuse me," I interrupted. "The woman sitting next to me is blind. Did you know that?"

"No," she answered.

"And the woman seated there, she's a hemophiliac. Did you know that?"

"No," she acknowledged.

"Well, then don't stand there and presume to know just by looking that everyone here in this room is 'so healthy' and therefore won't cost much to care for. You can't tell from simply looking at someone how healthy or not they are, or how their circumstances might change in the blink of an eye forcing them to receive more costly care."

Afterwards, I told her to go back and tell the Clintons that she wasn't the appropriate person to be speaking at these events, which she didn't like but it was true. She had neither the life experience nor qualifying knowledge of her audience to have been in the room.

Dick had worked tirelessly with me to formulate the bones, if you will, of RTK. Over the next six months Citizens for the Right to Know formalized to a full coalition.

Kassy Perry, founder of Sacramento's Perry Communications, Inc. (recognized today as a leader among PR firms nationally experienced in the health care arena) was an expert in both strategy and messaging—the art of building the pathways necessary to achieve heightened consumer awareness and ultimately, influence policy.

Kassy was committed to helping us build RTK as a consumer educational initiative with far-reaching goals and began giving life to Dick's vision and structure—refining the infrastructure, expanding the coalition's membership, and implementing outreach goals that could build consensus and alter the trajectory of managed care in terms of disclosure laws. Renee Paper from Nevada, Hemophilia Foundation of Nevada, and Laura Mitchell from the MS Society also joined our core team.

Kassy and I became the spokespersons for the group, Kassy taking lead during those times in which a professional representative was appropriate, while I continued to represent the face and stories of "the patient."

While I had become accustomed to speaking in public, I had, to date, been dragging the same "passionate, but angry" hairdresser/advocate to all my appearances, but something more, something smarter was now necessary.

Kassy, in her efforts to position us before larger, more influential decision makers, began to guide me in the art of maintaining a strong, undeniable, and passionate message while at the same time, leaving my more confrontational and angry persona at the door. I needed to grow as a speaker who could engage the willing (and non-willing) in the notion that advocating for the rights of patients was the right thing to do on many levels. I needed to learn how to communicate in a calm, policy-educated, and smart manner to outline the unacceptable state quo while also demonstrating the viable means and ways to changing it and how they (their agency, association or professional organization) could help make that change possible.

With Kassy helping me with, my transformation as a speaker (however doubtful I was at the time) quickly took shape, along with a significant rise in my confidence. I was still "me," only better equipped to step onto any field of play before any audience, knowing that my message was respectful, coherent, and that I had right on my side. But more so, I was able to formulate that message within the context of what my audience cared about, which varied from group to group. The end game was always clear: define the terms by which doing the right thing by consumers would produce a win for all concerned. Such appearances may have happened on someone else's home turf (a small association gathering, larger conference, or the state legislature), but with help from Kassy, I owned the field when I was done.

Kassy also taught me that defining and delivering an effective message didn't have to be complicated, and in fact, the simpler the better. A great example was when Kassy appeared before the state legislature and held up a small bag of potato chips on behalf of better disclosure within health plans. "Why is it," she questioned, "that we know more about what's in this product than we do about our health plans?"

She also used the example of purchasing a new car for which the sticker on the inside of the window tells you everything you need to know about that model, including mileage. Not so, however, with the typical health plan. In hindsight, during an interview for this book, Kassy referred to it as the "apple pie and motherhood" of messaging…what no one could argue with!

As it had happened before, RTK and my evolving relationship with Kassy was about to springboard into something even better that would allow me to reach new horizons and new levels of advocacy. Pinch me, someone!

CHAPTER 9

Executive Hair Stylist Takes on Managed Care

They say that before evolution, comes revolution. I believe that.

Now, revolutions are not always won or lost among the masses or even visible at all to those around us, but whether personal or professional, on behalf of many or a few, something somewhere has to give for change to occur.

In hindsight, Citizens for the Right to Know was indeed a revolution—a coming together of many on behalf of all concerned for change. But I think if you spoke to the individuals involved, you'd learn that for each, a personal revolution was occurring simultaneously. Funny how that works…the timing, the fateful events, the circumstances that drive us into unfamiliar places. That was certainly true in my story.

There comes a time in everyone's life where you suddenly realize you've outgrown your familiar, safe, and comfortable day-to-day shoes.

Some refer to such moments as milestones of sorts, much like when you realized as a young adult that being 100 percent responsible for yourself was going to be a lot harder than you thought, or when you catch yourself echoing the words of your own mother for the first time—reciting one of those deplorable lines you swore you would never say to your own children.

We do as we know, right? That is, until we know better.

I had learned more about myself and the world around me in the short span of seven years than I had racked up in all of my adult life. While I'm grateful to all my early lessons and those that (for good or bad) played an important role, the shift in me was, at times, unrecognizable. But it was nevertheless undeniable.

As time and my efforts on behalf of the TMJ Society marched on, the life I once knew was slipping further and further into the past.

First to come are the challenges that test your mettle and, little by little, expand your capacity to grow. Old belief systems (about yourself and others) transform almost unconsciously until one day, it becomes clear that there's no turning back.

While those old, comfortable shoes have defined you in so many ways and served you well…molded to fit perfectly until now, suddenly you're stepping to a new tune with different terrain beneath you. And don't look now, but you're actually running! Me…running? Why, yes! I am running! Who would have ever thought…and look at how fast I'm going!

By this time, my career in cosmetology had spanned nearly thirty years. I had built a successful business, nearly lost it all, and then rebuilt it even stronger than before. But now the question was, "Is my heart still in it?" Was it possible to put the genie back in the bottle and return to my old routine surrounded, arguably, by the safety of willfully ignorant bliss and blind faith?

The salon was more than just a place that provided for me financially. It's where some of my most enduring relationships began. It was a place where I played a starring role in the happiness of others, helping them feel attractive and confident. It was also a place where, for the most part, I knew the rules, the acceptable best practices, and even more so, I was in control.

Yet, the world, as I had come to experience it, was much, much bigger, and the idea that my role in it could be even bigger was too much to ignore. The endless possibilities of what I might achieve if I had more time to devote to the TMJ Society and patient advocacy took center stage in my mind. I needed to make some decisions.

I decided to sell the salon to one of my hairdressers and his wife, which allowed me a more flexible schedule and the ability to maintain my usual clientele (and income) without the responsibility of the salon's overall operation.

More and more, Kassy Perry was asking me to testify on various pieces of California legislation as either a patient with a story to tell, the founder of the TMJ Society, or as a representative of Citizens for the Right to Know. Sometimes all three! I was becoming well-known around the Capitol (some say infamous!) and respect for my testimony as a patient advocate grew. More and more, I began to see my own career path having a direct link to Kassy and thus began to badger her about putting me on staff at Perry Communications.

Kassy had begun to realize that she needed me full time as well, but how to structure our work together financially without jeopardizing my independence with the TMJ Society or RTK would take some thoughtful discussion.

Kassy remembers, "There wasn't any more money within the administrative-only grants available to us for RTK to bring Liz on full time at the firm. So we—Liz and I—had to envision more of a new role for her at my firm based on what we were learning in the field, the world in which patients and those who cared for them actually lived."

Mind you, I had never worked in an office environment before and knew absolutely nothing about computers. Still, the thought of working full time with Kassy was exciting, and it wasn't long before we had a plan that allowed me to make the leap. I was no longer "the hairdresser."

"I was developing other health care and pharmaceutical clients that could benefit from someone like Liz out in the field doing outreach efforts," Kassy recalled. "On their behalf, Liz would spend four days a week speaking to patients, providers, health organizations, and so on, helping to develop educational campaigns and legislative wording in cooperation with like-minded groups and/or clients.

"While only one day a week was specifically devoted to RTK, the relationships and contacts she was fostering as a member of Perry Communications also served the larger goals and influence of RTK.

It was perfect and also allowed RTK, as well as the TMJ Society to maintain, both financially and in terms of an agenda, independence from our client base."

As Outreach Coordinator for Perry Communications and their many clients, I began to build a gold mine—a database of advocacy groups, experts, lawmakers, and their staff, as well as other stakeholders within health care that RTK would have access to. Likewise, my work in the field would often bring about the discovery of problems experienced by patients, physicians, or other care providers. We could see healthcare trends beginning to emerge and strategize on how to ensure access and disclosure was always on the forefront, putting patients first.

With every new campaign, we broadened our exposure to the media as well as the public, strengthening our understanding of the health care landscape, the power brokers that controlled it, and those who were suffering as a direct result. It was an amazing time in which we also helped to develop other advocacy groups regarding lesser known illnesses.

Kassy summed it up perfectly, "Precisely because of our work in the field with patients and advocacy groups, we were finding out in real time what needed to be done, what's working, and what's not, and we began bridging those gaps."

We were creating not only the space for that work, but bringing the conversations themselves out into the light of day. Furthermore, we had to figure out common ground between stakeholders, build upon individual ideas in a way that no matter what the opposing agendas were overall, everyone could agree upon something. Change, I discovered, can only happen *after* some type of shift occurs, no matter how small.

Understanding this was not only vital to our efforts then; it continues to be of even greater importance today if we are to overcome the challenges we face in health care.

As Kassy recalls, "We had to decided what we could live with and what we couldn't. More so, we had agreed to respectfully disagree with others and put aside some opposing points of conflict [historical/political philosophy] regarding certain organizations in order to foster instead, viewpoints that we knew both sides could in fact agree on and work towards effectively."

In some cases, it meant walking into what many would consider enemy territory.

> Liz was fearless when it came to entering the lion's den…literally defying them to bring political or other opposing agendas into the conversation. Most advocates tend to "stick to their own" in an attempt to force change from a safe, collective corner of strength. Believe me, it doesn't exist. Strength in numbers is one thing, but eventually, you have to meet with the other side. Liz and I wouldn't play that way. Liz could respectfully speak with anyone, and from her informed, kind position, foster those ideas that anyone should want to engage, regardless. It's still her strength today and why she can move the ball in ways that others can't.

Warren Barnes, former legal counsel for the California Department of Managed Health Care, is correct when he says, "Everyone sincerely likes Liz. I don't think I've ever heard anyone speak badly about her personally, regardless who they represent."

Knowing your perceived antagonist and navigating that mine field was one thing, but sometimes it was just as difficult for us to identify our friends.

Early on, HMOs had already begun to screw the consumer and had moved on to squeezing the physicians as part of their cost-savings plan but had not yet begun sticking it to the pharmaceutical companies. We knew, however, it was only a matter of time.

Our work with RTK regarding disclosure of drug formularies was angering the HMO lobbyists, who in turn were making life difficult for the pharmaceutical lobbyist, and they were quick to unload a little of their pain on us.

Some pharmaceutical companies were still trying to negotiate for contracts that would include their drugs on the various HMO drug formularies and saw our efforts on behalf of consumers as an obstruction for them. The pharmaceutical lobbyists saw the HMOs as their friends and customers, but we knew then, as is still the case, that if the health plans could figure out a way to exclude paying for newer more expensive drugs, they would. What we didn't know back then was just how quickly that was going to happen, no matter how far the pharmaceutical companies bent over for them.

Eventually, our prediction of the real impact HMOs would have on the availability of drugs within their individual formularies became a reality...so too a little more respect for our efforts from some in the pharmaceutical industry itself.

We had begun a significant campaign designed for open enrollment periods that encouraged employees to ask questions about promised coverage and, specifically, questions relating to what drugs were included in their formularies. Our messaging was going out to both employees and company executives who were responsible for deciding which plans to make available.

During an upcoming open enrollment, we were leaked the new (and altered) drug formulary of PacificCare, now part of UnitedHealth, which we devoured line by line and compared it to the policy currently in force but about to expire.

Under the current rules, an HMO didn't have to disclose such changes. Instead, an unsuspecting employee would learn that they no longer had coverage for his/her medications until long after signing on the dotted line for another year...when it was too late to change their mind and choose another plan.

The document exposed the fact that a health plan was dropping entire classes of drugs, including antidepressants or supplementing some drugs with others that were (arguably) less effective for some people or perhaps more cost-effective drugs. For the patient suffering from mental illness who had finally found stability on a particular drug, having to change drugs—or worse, finding out no drugs in a particular class were covered—could be devastating.

If HMOs weren't going to be required to share such information, we were going to do it ourselves.

Again, our job wasn't to dictate what drugs should be covered or advocate for a specific brand. Our demand was for disclosure of any changes to a formulary and to level the playing field to ensure patients received the access they and their employers assumed they were paying for.

We took out full-page ads, cosponsored by NAMI (National Alliance of Mental Illness) in *The Los Angeles Times* and others exposing the new, untold formulary changes and how patients with mental health concerns could be affected. The *Times* pulled the ad and refused to run it, going so far as to have their legal counsel call us to inform us of their decision. Further, they noted that PacificCare was a huge advertiser with the *Times* and felt our ad to be irresponsible.

Shortly afterward, we were also contacted by the legal counsel of PacificCare who threatened to sue Kassy, myself, and RTK unless we pulled the ads.

In the context of a tense phone confrontation, Kassy asked again and again for the representative to tell us what in the ad was not factual, but they couldn't.

Under great duress, Kassy called NAMI to update them on the situation. We knew we were right, but still, our reputations and livelihoods were on the line, not to mention that of RTK.

Finally, we got the break we needed when Kassy received a call from the top legal firm in Washington, DC, who did pro bono work for NAMI. The attorney said, "Go ahead…Run the ad! We'll cover any and all legal fees necessary to defend it." Further, they implied that they'd love nothing more than to have the publicity of PacificCare suing one the largest grass roots mental health organization in the country. Bring it!

As quickly as possible, we called the *Orange County Register* and told them the whole story. They loved it and ran a front-page story the next day including how the *Times* had bowed to pressure from their advertiser.

Rough times, we kept on pins and needles and didn't know who all our friends were.

Was it any wonder that, not being sure who our friends were at times, we often felt suspicious of events that coincided with our campaigns? Kassy's car got keyed, and my tires were slashed. Were these events related? Probably not. But in the heat of things, we lived on pins and needles more than was comfortable.

Thankfully, the times in between were more rewarding and lifted our spirits. It was also fun.

My nature is to engage in friendly chatter with just about anyone I meet, and that served me well during those years. Time and again, it seemed like divine fate would sit me next to someone important on a plane or find myself having breakfast in a hotel I was staying as Colin Powell in Washington, DC, or someone with the most amazing story or connection that would later serve our efforts. I would return home literally giddy with incredible stories, hardly believable, actually! There were times I couldn't believe I was being paid to do what I was doing!

Still, each and every trip home was a return to reality and usually more evidence that we had a long, long way to go.

Gag orders became a huge issue, especially as it related to treatments and medications not covered in the health plans. Quite literally, there were three people in the physician's exam room—the physician, the patient, and an HMO ensuring that the physician purposefully withheld information about available treatments from their patients.

Within the contracts between the HMO and medical providers, physicians were forbidden to speak to patients about treatments and medications that weren't covered by the HMO, no matter the value of the treatment or drug. Physicians were struggling with the restrictive policies and largely remained silent out of fear they would be booted from the plans.

Members of the medical community began to "leak" information about such policies to us, and we, in turn, began to fight back on behalf of patients and their right to have all pertinent medical information available disclosed.

Were we puppets of the CMA? Certainly not, but they understood what our success on behalf of patients would mean to their physicians and supported our efforts, even if behind closed doors early on.

We worked with Assembly member Martin Gallegos, chair of the Assembly Health Committee and State Senator Diane Watson, chair of the Senate Health Committee, on legislation banning gag rules regarding treatments or medications not covered.

I'd like to say that times have changed. But when it comes to drugs, today's physicians are so beaten down by the whole process of formularies, prior approval, and communication with the health plans (that seemingly go into a deep dark hole) that many will offer whatever meek excuse necessary to encourage a patient to accept—gracefully—whatever drug is easily covered. "They're all the same... really," seems to be easy enough to offer up as an excuse. It's not true. But it's "true enough" for most physicians to get their job done without added frustration.

While many rail against the idea of government involvement in health care choices, they fail to understand that corporate America beat them into the exam room by a mile and then some, a long time ago, and have little intention of leaving anytime soon.

As a member-funded coalition—not a non-profit, but a network of non-profits—our goal at RTK was to work behind the scenes fostering education and legislation being sponsored by other, often larger organizations on behalf of California consumers. We were often accused of being a front group for the California Medical Association (CMA) or PhRMA, the drug maker's lobbying wing. But it simply was not true, and we worked hard to maintain our distinction. If, for example, consumers could evaluate a health plan and determine what was covered and what wasn't, including the drugs on a particular formulary, they could decide for themselves which plan to accept.

Our goal at RTK was to ensure that HMOs were required to disclose what drugs were and weren't on their formularies and that physicians had the freedom to speak about and prescribe whatever medication they felt was appropriate for the patient. RTK did not take a stand on, or represent in any fashion, one drug over another. Kassy was raised within a family of medical providers, her father a physician and cancer researcher and her mother a nurse. She felt very strongly, as did I, that it was important for patients to get the right drug the first time and that nobody else, such as the HMO, should be in that discussion.

Likewise, in regards to the CMA or our local/state medical society, what was good for patients was usually good for their physician members. Some within the medical community often fed us information about what was happening to patients or how their physicians were being restricted, such as with the gag rules, when they themselves were powerless to do anything about it. They often helped to support or validate what was happening on the ground and/or helped put us in contact with patients for their stories, but nothing more. Certainly, the CMA never contributed to RTK financially.

As we waited for and continued to work toward strong disclosure laws, we had to engage in…let's say…creative action, for lack of a better term.

Initially, HMOs saw a huge opening in the senior market—the space between traditional Medicare supplemental insurance policies and the later-termed Medicare advantage programs.

Individual HMO plans would sponsor widely advertised benefit events for seniors in Sacramento and other communities, offering free eyeglass repair kits and more in exchange for sitting through their product offering.

Kassy and I would show up, sit in back of the room and proceed to ask question after question to their frustration. We'd ask what senior consumers *should* be asking but didn't know they needed to. Eventually, the HMO representatives would figure out what we were doing—exposing their plans for what they were and what they lacked—and with that, they would ask us to leave. We knew we had done a good job and touched some nerves when we got kicked out.

But we couldn't be everywhere at once, so we also went to work creating a storehouse of information that consumers could access 24-7. We offered online resources for patients who felt they had been abused by the system or didn't know where to turn for advice.

We created a website to help patients understand the maze of coverage options and created pamphlets (still available online today—and still applicable) with titles such as, "Choices: What You Need to Know" and "California's Emerging Advocate: You!"

We also designed a "shop around" report card on prescription drugs to help patients compare drug costs in the US with those in Canada and even produced a video on advocacy.

Our success began to get noticed in other states too. Soon, I was traveling to Colorado, Oregon, Arizona, and Washington to help organize and set up coalitions like RTK in those states as well.

One of our most successful outreach campaigns was called "HMO! Oh, No!" which helped to identify HMO horror stories and find victims of HMO abuses. The public could identify with the stories, the faces and the families affected by such abuse.

It's nearly impossible to convey how proud I was of some of our campaigns and the Continuity of Care Bill fits that description. RTK supported the passage of Assembly Bill 974, which ensured continuity of care by requiring health plans to pay for treatments for preexisting medical conditions if drugs previously prescribed were dropped from their formularies. If you were an existing HMO plan member on a particular drug before the formulary changed, you could remain on that drug and have it covered. The passage of AB 974 affected countless thousands of California health care consumers.

RTK, not having any particular horse in the race when it came to drugs, but more so, advocating that the right drugs should always be made available, also joined the fight against Kaiser's efforts to block Viagra as a covered drug since many patients suffered from injuries or chronic conditions that impeded normal erectile function. In some cases, drugs taken for a nonrelated health condition were responsible for making Viagra necessary.

When Claritin, a widely prescribed nonsedating antihistamine went over-the-counter, we led the effort to prevent health plans from dropping the entire "non-sedating" class from their formularies, as Claritin alone didn't work for everyone and shouldn't dictate an entire class. For those who were prescribed different medication from the same class, they still needed their medications covered, as they weren't always able to take the new, over-the-counter and cheaper Claritin. And of course, we helped pass two Assembly bills increasing mental health parity funding and increasing access to treatment for mental health consumers, which made unrestricted access to proper treatment and drugs more widely available.

Yes, I wanted to do more when faced with the decision to sell the salon, or not…or to go to work for Kassy full time, or not. I wanted more personally and professionally, and I got it. But along the way, I also achieved more than I could have ever dreamed possible with a little help from my friends, my family, and my partners in advocacy.

Of course, none of it would have been possible without the faith and trust Kassy placed in me. There are not enough pages to tell all the individual stories of those I met along the way, but suffice to say, they know my gratitude for all their help and patience, and they know too that their investment in me lives on for battles yet to come.

I love the energy of Washington, DC—the people, the power, and the sheer importance of it all.

From outside the Beltway, it's easy to thrive on a steady diet of cynicism, but once within the halls of American history, a sense of majesty and principle—that which our country was founded on—overshadows all else.

That I would find myself here, testifying before a congressional body that had the power to correct wrongs and alter the course of health care delivery with their decisions, was surreal. It was the ultimate (dream) achievement in discovering my voice and developing it to the degree that my thoughts, opinions, and experience now would become part of congressional record. My words, and those of countless, otherwise average Americans before me, cannot be erased or ignored as our country progresses. How can I not hold something like that dear?

Were it not for the tremendous weight of responsibility I felt—knowing that the U.S. Senate's decisions, based at least in part on my testimony, could further infringe on the rights of patients, or enhance the quality of care received—my feet might not have ever touched the floor. But I carried with me to Washington every patient I had ever met who suffered and every member organization involved with RTK, knowing that they were all depending on me to deliver for them. My voice had to represent them all, clearly, effectively and passionately.

Twice I've had the honor of testifying before the United States Congress, both before subcommittees dealing with health care.

My first visit to Washington was in 1999 shortly after joining Perry Communications to testify before the Senate's Special Committee on Aging.

The U.S. Government Accounting Office was looking into formulary practices in California: the bedrock of some of my work with Citizens for the Right to Know.

Within my testimony, I spoke to the unregulated, arbitrary, and make-it-up-as-you-go- policies of the health plans, patient hardship, and/or negative outcomes be damned.

I discussed the bait-and-switch tactics used by health plans in which different brands (often cheaper, older, or generic drugs) were arbitrarily substituted for more expensive name brands. I discussed the lack of fundamental patient rights when it came to formularies: disclosure regarding coverage, continuity of care, the impact of formularies regarding decisions that were made between a patient and their physician.

I also testified to the patterns of denial often plaguing the system—that a plan could drop a drug for any reason without notice or, worse, deny coverage spanning a whole class of drugs all together without concern or consideration as to the adverse risks (negative impact) it would have on patients.

I was excited to testify before this Senate committee because I knew that the problems plaguing California were happening in other states as well. It was an opportunity to take our message national, to influence patient rights, and to further access to the medications they needed in all states. It was also important due to the expanded role of independent Medicare supplemental and Medicare "advantage" policies within the HMO industry, which were growing in number and concern over Part D cost factors.

Just a year later, my second visit to Congress before the Senate's Committee on Health, Education, Labor, and Pensions involved prescription drug prices. It was my testimony then, and my continued belief today, that any "huge rise" in prescription drug prices was a facade created by the health plans—a red herring designed to restrict the market in their favor. I testified to the long and effective competitive nature of pharmaceuticals and the need for consumers to shop around as they do with other basic items of need. Prescription drug costs varied widely from one drug store to the next, with the greatest cost savings found within larger chains with national purchasing power. In many cases, the savings touted by those traveling to Canada could be realized here at home given some consumer-savvy diligence.

Senate committee hearings often contain two opposing sides to an issue, or at the very least, two opposing influences having some effect on commerce—one way or the other. But each time I sat down before the Senate panel, I did so on behalf of a third, and arguably the most important entity often overshadowed during debates of policy…consumers of health care…patients.

My intent was to ensure that no matter the finger-pointing, no matter the preponderance of lobbyists, the outcome in policy would protect health care consumers and put the best interests of the physician-patient relationship ahead of all others.

And judging by the results, the notion that an individual has no role to play in today's government, or no voice in the direction of our country, is simply not true. My testimony, my voice on behalf of health care consumers, counted and played a significant role in achieving the outcome we all sought.

I remember like it was yesterday, the day I entered the Capitol after my presentation at NIH when I nearly felt faint as I watched the Senate debate issues, and I had to leave quickly. I didn't know then what my mission would be. I didn't know what message I would bring to Congress. I just knew I would have one. That all changed the day I testified. Now my mission clearer than ever. I knew why I had gone through all I did early on when I was denied care for my TMJ. I knew now that my voice mattered, and people were listening. I knew that bigger changes were coming and that I would have a part in that change.

CHAPTER 11

Lessons from the Hair Salon:
Roots and Grassroots

You might be surprised to learn that understanding a patient's rights and advocating for those rights is a lot like working as a stylist in a multi-service salon.

It's all in the nuances of unspoken language; the relationship between who they really are and who they want to be perceived to be; and of course, the subtleties of change.

Any good stylist will tell you that it takes time and effort to develop a good working relationship with a new customer. You need to get to know them, determine their hair type, their style preferences, and their lifestyle and work routines.

You need to take a moment to observe their color choices of hair and clothing. Is there a pattern? And you must consider the whole person—their skin tone and facial structure. How do they carry themselves?

Some characteristics, with time and experience, are relatively quick to decipher. Others are detected only through subtle clues, followed by discussion.

The correct hair color, for example, can inject life and vibrancy into otherwise common or dull locks. Along with the right cut, it can provide the appearance of added volume and nurtured health, where beforehand boredom and dread resided.

Incorrect color can make someone look tired and washed and even enhance the appearance of bags under the eyes!

Hues and other subtleties of color can be broken down into basic molecular structures, something I wanted my customers to understand. Mixing color is both a science and an art, and I wanted clients to see how color could change not only their hair, but their personality, affecting how they viewed themselves and indeed how others viewed them as well.

Color also changes when the mixture was allowed to cool down, something else to keep in mind when designing a change for a client.

There were many steps to ensuring a perfect blend and beautiful outcome…a beautiful whole.

Consider, if you will, that given the number of salons throughout the state of California, all using (for the most part) the same general color products, each blending color bases in their own unique way. Yet not every stylist will produce the same result. Each, in fact has his or her biases regarding current trends and personal tastes—personal methods, likes and dislikes, as well as work ethics—that are blended in as well.

In California, there's no shortage of hair stylists, nor is there a shortage of patient advocates. But just as I had my own style as a… well, stylist, I also have my own style as an advocate, and almost no one does it same way I do.

As a health care advocate, you could say that I operated much the same as I did as a stylist. I took the time necessary to get to know whom I was dealing with, whether it was a patient, a health plan, a legislator, or fellow advocacy organization.

I studied all for clues to their nature, their position, and what their motivating factors were: profit, pension, or passion? Were they decision makers or well-intended grunts without the power to negotiate in good faith? Were they industry leaders or followers?

What was their stake in the game, and was I seeing the real person or entity, or just the face that one puts on for public display… different, of course, from the one they wear in the board room?

And just like the pros and cons of hair color, did their position in the industry give them that certain bounce that comes with expressed compassion and dedication followed by action, or did they appear tired—tired of the schemes, tired of the resistance, tired of playing the role of the enforcer of bad and disheartening news: "We're denying your coverage."

Were their words spoken with confidence and strength, or did their body language give them up as being less than genuine, playing the role as best they could.

Most of the time, I looked for one thing—the blink. That moment when I could tell that there's room, no matter how small, to find common ground…a place to begin and a place to grow from.

Patience, persistence, and perseverance are the virtues of a successful advocate—the ability to be strong in conviction, yet flexible, respectful, and appreciative.

Perhaps because I came to patient advocacy as a patient first, a consumer injured by the same system that was supposed to protect patients, I begin every issue from the patient's perspective.

What patients are most likely to be affected by a specific health care policy?

Once I determined that, I'd speak with them first, then learn all that I can about their illness, their health plans, how they've suffered, and what they've done to get better.

While the individual diagnosis may differ, as well as their health plan, far too often the story is the same—a losing battle shrouded in deception, lack of access, or unjustified denial.

My next stop is to chat with any advocacy or educational organization involved with the specific nature of the disease itself. They know where the road blocks exist in policy— where the bodies are, as it were. They know the players on the inside track, as well as the gatekeepers whose job it is to run interference and ensure you go home defeated and reminded of your place.

My goal isn't to recreate the wheel but to form coalitions of people and organizations that together offer a larger, more inclusive and effective voice with the power of numbers and experience behind their message.

Like a new customer in the salon, learning the subtleties of stakeholders on any given health issue takes time. You must build individual relationships that can carry you the distance required, as change doesn't happen quickly or without great effort.

Certainly, there are those rare occasions in which simple reasoning ("This is better for patients and their health outcomes") works like a charm, and all minds can agree. But in truth, those cases are the exception, not the rule.

More often than not, change that benefits patients will often come at a price, at least on the front end of costs, that can't be offset by "reasoning" and arguments regarding best practices. Because the right thing to do also comes with a price tag, one must be able to show the reduced cost overall when patient outcomes are better, and health, in the long term, is considered.

And because (initially) the more costly "right thing to do" runs counter to any corporation's fiduciary responsibility to its investors and stockholders, state, and federal government regulations must often intercede on the consumer's behalf through regulation.

Such regulations are not meant to stifle a free marketplace or impede in any way on the profits of an insurance company but rather ensure that when the choice is clearly the health and well-being of the consumer versus the profit of the industry, patients are the first concern.

Interestingly enough, although rarely brought to the forefront of discussion, doing right by patients is profitable. As is often the case with preventative measures and has been proven over and over, doing right by patients is extremely cost effective in the long run, benefiting the bottom line of all stakeholders over time.

True advocacy isn't about backroom deals with one player out of the many. It's about changing the culture and environment of health care and providing the best outcome for patients.

I'm not about putting Band-Aids on bursting dams and short fixes. They never work. Instead, I take on worthy battles for the long haul, understanding that my best path to success is by forming coalitions of like-minded people and organizations, and that my commitment will require many months, if not years, of hard work, one small victory at a time.

Advocacy also requires strength of purpose—the ability to clearly and effectively define what your work is about and what it's not.

Citizens for the Right to Know, as it grew in both membership and public awareness, was exposed to many needs and hardships felt within the patient community. As each would pull at our heartstrings, it was necessary—imperative, in fact—that we remain focused on our primary mission: patient rights as it pertained to disclosure of, and access to, coverage within health plans.

Individually, members, including myself (as the founder of the TMJ Society), could assist or join other coalitions whose purpose of advocacy and goals were different, but RTK held to its initial purpose. To do otherwise would have diluted our energy, our efforts, and eventually, our outcomes. Remaining true to our purpose meant every win was like collecting another power tool in our armory, each one furthering our voice and strength in California's policy community, as both drivers of consumer-centered disclosure policy and patient rights.

When the consumer disclosure goals of RTK were met, we celebrated all we had accomplished and graciously disbanded…each member returning to the needs of their individual organization, and/or regrouping with other coalitions to further progressive inroads to better access and quality of care.

It doesn't mean you simply quit, but you do recognize when it's time to take what you've learned and apply it elsewhere. We won the "right to know" for citizens, and it was time to spread my wings in other worthy ventures within health care advocacy.

It was time to reassess what I had learned and the relationships I had built. What strengths did I now possess that I could put to better use? What role could I play in the still-evolving world of health care access and how could that role benefit consumers?

As it turned out, my work and all the success that followed was prelude for what was still to come.

I know! Can you imagine my world getting even bigger and better?

CHAPTER 12

The Advocate in You

Writer Tom Wolfe dubbed the 1970s as "the me decade."

Some people think that today, people are more selfish than ever. Certainly the way in which many important issues are framed politically makes it easy to let cynicism take the lead and agree that ours is a public that has lost its *humane* way.

But look around and you'll find a country in which people, by and large, continue to put the health and well-being of others first.

I've traveled around the world to military bases and have seen extraordinary men and women who are willing to sacrifice for their families and, in some cases, their lives for the good of their country. My son, Matt, has served in the armed forces for over two decades, and I am so proud of his service to our country.

I see great sacrifice in our post-baby boom generation, the "sandwich generation" whose members often care for both their parents and their children. They are enormously concerned about today's quality of life and care deeply about the salvation of our world.

And a great many of those I've worked with over the years have contributed greatly for no reason other than because they could. They worked within specific and often for-profit health-access industries and knew they could help bridge the gaps. They knew that it was not only the right thing to do but was also good for business and their industry, despite the corporate heads that often fought us. Many did so in secret, risking their careers and their family's security in the process.

So what makes a good advocate? Do they simply "care" more than others?

Hardly.

Most health care advocates I meet are just like you and me: average Joes or Janes that found themselves in the throes of a health care delivery system that, in most cases, either failed them personally or failed someone they love.

Many have become involuntary stakeholders, diagnosed personally (or someone they love…a spouse, parent, or child) with an illness for which our system of delivery falls short, or worse, fails to deliver at all.

For others, what began as nothing more than a job—a place of employment or professional outreach—grew into something that touched their soul and offered unexpected commitment, that special "feels like I've come home" sense of purpose.

People get involved for many personal reasons, but they all have something in common: they want to make things better, whether you're talking expanded choice and/or access to care, affordability, consumer rights, disclosure and/or education, or better quality of patient outcomes.

All have a singular motive: the desire to help those who are not in the position to help themselves.

The wonderful thing about advocacy is that the only certificate required is the one that deems you *human*. You don't need a college degree or proven professional accomplishment, just the heart of a lion and a commitment liken to that of a mother bear to her cubs.

You choose…Your voice either matters or it doesn't. And once you make that choice, the "how to and where?" details will begin to fall into place naturally.

You've heard the notion that if you buy a red car, suddenly you see red cars everywhere! Well, the same is true for advocacy. The opportunity to expand your capacity to help people is everywhere.

You can be at the grocery store, the gas station, your own doctor's office, or on the phone with a friend, and people who either need your assistance, know someone who needs your assistance, or can offer *you* assistance through their own contacts suddenly appear in your path.

Articles begin to catch your attention in the newspaper or on a social network or blog site. The more you share your own story and interest in change, the more others share stories of their own or the stories of someone they know.

There's no shortage of organizations already formed that would either welcome your involvement, or could, perhaps, join a coalition of your own making to expand your efforts through a more collective voice.

And while it's true that today, I wear many hats—secretary, grant writer, key negotiator, community outreach coordinator—and perform duties ranging from founder and president to accounting, it didn't begin that way. I had a lot of help from others with personal strengths and professional skills in areas that I lacked.

My journey began as one, and an injured "one" at that, with others lending their time, skills and experience to benefit not only my situation, but the needs of many like me.

Speaking up and speaking out is a process.

As you begin, don't try to conquer the world overnight.

Believe me, I understand how passion and a search for justice and purpose can overwhelm your every thought and keep you up at night, mulling over the hurdles and possibilities. But before you become sleep deprived and a stranger to your family, consider the following first steps:

- Define your purpose. When you can narrow that defini-tion to one sentence, you're ready to move on.
- Define your mission. What actions must take place in order to bring about meaning change?
- Define who is adversely affected: Is it a select group of individuals or are there cross-segments of society involved, and if so, how do they connect?
- Define your personal story and how it represents the expe-rience of others affected by the same issue. Get to the meat of your story and stick to it, as it will define your testi-

mony in a meaningful way or create lingering doubts with those who could help carry your message forward if it's changing over time (media, experts, other advocates, etc).

- Define your strengths and weaknesses. What personal experience or abilities do you bring to the party that can help construct an aggressive and competent campaign? This can be your own compelling story, your professional organizational skills, your ability to communicate effectively, or even your nature as a hub—the person who others (family, friends) have always turned to and have been able to count on when the chips were down. Life experience counts as much as any other in the world of advocacy.

Remember, I owned and managed a successful salon—hardly the background one considers to be destined to testify before the US Congress!

In fact, Warren Barnes, now retired, of the California Department of Managed Health Care put it this way.

> If Liz had a business degree or some other higher education credentials, she would have most definitely gone to work in some professional capacity for the state, and ultimately would have been far less effective and successful as part of the very system she was trying to change. The fact that she was representing consumers of health care (from the outside of that system) in the capacity of a patient with a personal story to tell, as well as diligent advocate who could present her case to anyone, served her and consumers well. She offered a voice and perspective that only someone on the outside of the system could, without a professional agenda or job to protect.

Be clear and honest with yourself. There were no advocacy groups for TMJ when I began; thus, it was necessary to create my own foundation, but you don't have to begin at the deep end of the pool.

There's a bounty of ways in which you can get involved and make a tremendous difference, no matter the issue. Consider the benefits of joining a local coalition with like-minded goals before setting out to change the world on your own. You'll learn the ropes, make some great contacts, and should you decide to break out on your own, you'll have a better idea of the landscape before you.

Above all, remember that even those who stanchly oppose you aren't your enemy. You simply haven't found the needle in the haystack yet…the one key issue or need that you both share and could develop together, if not now, someday. Bridges are to be crossed, not burned.

CHAPTER 13

That's Not What I Said: Working with the Media

When it comes to speaking with the media and giving interviews, there are three rules you *must* remember:

> There's no such thing as "off the record."
> There's no such thing as "off the record."
> There's no such thing as "off the record."

Above all else, reporters are looking for a story, and if you don't define yours, they'll be happy to do it for you.

Over the course of my career as an advocate, I've had both good and bad encounters with journalists, a term I'll use respectfully here. Some of my finest affiliations with the press were with the *San Francisco Chronicle's* medical writers.

Not every reporter is jaded or lazy, and most will come prepared with background, but you should be ready with documentation and/ or easily verifiable facts to support your interview points. There are some wonderfully talented and caring writers out there who will work hard to make sure they get the story right.

By nature, I was rather trusting initially, assuming that reporters who called for an interview with me were interested in our mission and plight on behalf of health consumers.

I assumed they wanted to tell my story as a means to educate their readership regarding the issues and pitfalls for our struggling health care delivery system.

And yes, I assumed early on that they would acknowledge my passion and tell of the human tragedies occurring every day at the hands of HMOs.

What is it they say about assuming something?

Part of your responsibility is defining what the story is, and is not, about.

Interviews I gave as founder of the TMJ Society were about the struggles of patients with TMJ to receive prompt and appropriate care coverage. As part of the story, my personal plight as a patient who had been egregiously denied care that, according to my policies, I was covered to receive, was often included to put a human face on the issue. It was about the unnecessary and life-destroying consequences that patients like me were forced to endure through no fault of our own. And it was about an emerging insurance plan system that cared more about the bottom line than it did helping patients.

Later, as I became a spokesperson for Citizens for the Right to Know, it was about the need for full disclosure laws that would inform consumers of what they could expect from a plan before becoming a member (an outline of what was covered or not, including drugs) and their right to receive notice of changes to that plan before they were instituted.

But my story was not about the pros and cons of HMOs or why someone should choose a PPO or private insurance over the HMO plans that were gaining popularity with employers. Nor was it about how some might try to "game" the system or the private physician's struggle with a changing business environment.

These and other issues may have been a part of the broad discussion regarding health insurance and delivery of care overall, but they weren't the issues I was advocating, and to misrepresent them as such was wrong.

When I first began giving interviews, I was Liz Helms, the hairdresser with TMJ. Not long afterward, I became Liz Helms, founder of the TMJ Society, followed by Liz Helms, member of RTK (as founder of the TMJ Society), and lastly, a public relations executive for Perry Communications, known as their director of advocacy and outreach. By then, I had become what is commonly, although not necessarily affectionately referred to as, a "flak," someone representing a special interest.

The press is interested in accuracy. But they're also just as concerned with creating a story that is dramatic and engaging. If you've got something important to say, great, but otherwise…quick! Remember those posted signs at the zoo: "Don't feed the tigers!"

It's not necessary—or advisable—to comment on every issue a reporter calls you about.

Should you receive a request out of the blue and want to offer a comment or quote, ask if you can call them back in just a few minutes—"Five minutes, I promise!"—so that you can take a moment to compose a comment worth giving, one with purpose rather than off the cuff, and even then, make sure you understand the angle the reporter is writing about.

When reporters talk to you they want to know several things:

- Are you telling the truth?
- Do you have a special interest in the case?
- Can your facts be verified?

They're often interested in your opinion as much as facts, and when offered, opinions can be misrepresented if taken out of context, so be careful.

Before agreeing to an interview, you need to know several things about the reporter and the publication requesting to speak with you.

- Who are their readers?
- What's the underlying story they're writing and why did they select you for comment?
- Have they written any other articles about this issue, and if so, where can they be found for review? (Note: If available, *read them first.*)
- How did they find out about you?
- Will the article be print only or posted online?

- Will they be obtaining comments from anyone else for this article? If so, who?
- What, if any, research have they already done for the article?
- Search for and read other articles they've written in the past so that you're familiar with their style of reporting.
- Do they offer readers in-depth and/or fair insight to problems, or do their articles typically highlight the issues only and offer little more in the way of resources?
- Ask if you'll be able to link to their article online afterward and if reprints are available?

Once you've done your homework and ensured that they've done theirs, define the message you want their readership to take away from your comments. What's the point you most want to drive home, why should readers care (how does it affect them personally), and what can the readers do to protect themselves and their families. Where can readers obtain more information?

Define your message in as few words as possible and stick to that message. It's easy to be taken off message by a reporter, but you should resist that as much as possible.

If you're asked a question about something off-topic, or anything beyond the scope of what you were lead to believe the article is about specifically, reject the sense that you're somehow obligated to go there. Stick to the topic of the interview you granted, as you have no idea what context your side comments will be used. Simply and respectfully state that perhaps that would be a topic you could comment on at another time.

Never believe that "get to know you" banter or friendly chitchat before an interview begins (or ends) is off the record! Something said in jest or within the innocent atmosphere of a more casual discussion long after the interview is over will often find its way into the story—or become your highlighted quote—and could alter the article altogether, and not in a way you'll appreciate. Remember at all times that your work and reputation are on the line. Your reputation is your stock in trade. Don't do anything that can cloud it for the purpose of a story.

It's important to develop mutually beneficial relationships with the media. They can be of great service when it comes to helping you educate the public and release important information, but keep it professional, not personal.

If you believe that a reporter requesting an interview is after a story that misrepresents your goals, don't be afraid to turn it down. Trust your gut and look for another media source.

And finally, be yourself. Don't try to project a personality or a person (professional or otherwise) that you're not. With all this in mind, here's a list of rules that are found on a magnet near my desk… something I refer to often as a reminder:

1. Always tell the truth.
2. Always tell the truth (this bears repeating because it's so important).
3. Keep your message simple.
4. Take your time; don't be afraid of the "er" or pause.
5. Always ask to have a question repeated.
6. Even if you tell a reporter it's "off the record," there's no such thing.
7. If you don't know an answer, say so, and get back to the reporter.
8. Don't be afraid of the media.
9. Understand that they're people too who have a job and deadlines to meet.

Lastly, it's a good idea to begin creating a spreadsheet of contact information early on. Include members of the press that you've already spoken to or would like to speak with in the future.

If they've written an article that you found particularly suited toward your needs in style or content, include it on the spreadsheet for quick reference.

Jot down other articles or topics they've covered for quick reference down the road. When you have something to release or want to generate interest in something you're involved with, you'll have contacts ready at your fingertips! That alone is half the battle!

CHAPTER 14

Lessons from the Abyss

In the throes of a crisis, we find it hard to see beyond the unfairness of what's happening all around us and to us.

Our inability, it seems, to control collateral damage and regain a sense of power over our circumstances becomes all-consuming.

It's as if we're simply hanging on for dear life while riding some high-speed roller coaster that's looping through never-ending sharp curves upside down. As one curve ends, another soon begins before we can recover.

We become, in such a state, frozen: incapable of recognizing the landscape before us and incapable too, of moving forward through the fire.

Looking back at my life, I've learned some indelible lessons from my TMD illness.

When I was sick, everything in my life was slipping away: my business, my health, my relationships and marriage, and most of all, my self-worth…everything. I was in the deepest, darkest pit of my life.

It was, I suppose, natural to question what I had done to deserve all that was happening…and expected, I guess, to assume that I had made bad or selfish choices along the way creating a backlash of karma against me.

But I understand now that from within that pain—and I'm speaking both of physical and emotional pain—a truth emerged that I would have never before considered.

The truth is, had I not been forced to endure so much—years of physical pain, sorrow, and loss, and yes, the unfairness and the plight of an innocent victim—I would have never developed into the staunch, ever-committed advocate that I became.

Had I received only nominal, or at its worse, extended resistance by my HMO followed by some form of resolution, I would have gone about my life picking up where I left off and accepting—despite how unacceptable in truth, it was—the whole mess as something one must navigate within the corporate structures of a changing health insurance industry.

Had I not been pushed to the brink of complete mental and physical destruction, I may have never considered the plight of others, who, despite my own awful story, endured worse than me.

And while looking back, I can also clearly see the apex of divine intervention that brought others into my life, altering forever the direction my life would take as a result.

But it's also true that through my need, my story, and my willingness to get up each day and fight, they too were allowed to develop their own story, their own willingness to participate in life and their own ability to fight an injustice that existed, unabated, around them in their own lives.

Together, we participated diligently in the grand experiment called life, and enriched our own lives while enriching that of others.

Would it have been possible, I wonder, should any of the individuals involved—friend or foe—played a different role, or no role at all, for us to arrive at the same outcome? I doubt it, for even those whose goal it was to put obstacles in our way, or impede our efforts in some way, played a vital role in the outcome of events and our chosen path.

They say you can't change history, and honestly, all considered, I don't know that I would if I could.

I learned that no matter how bad it gets, how low you go, how hard you're hit by life, *never give up*. Ever.

The lessons indeed are in the journey, and every lesson carries forward something significant for journeys still to come. And let's be clear: your journey ends only with your last breath. Until then, each and every moment, be it joyful or painful, has meaning and purpose.

Along the way, I made some amazing discoveries about myself, including that I was stronger than I ever gave myself credit for.

Before my illness, my singular goal in life, and thus my day-to-day choices involved taking care of my family, their needs and wants. In short, I lived to make my family and others happy, rarely thinking about myself.

I also did what I needed to do to survive and, in hindsight, not much more. Even voting didn't matter to me, as like everything else. I couldn't see the immediate or long-term influence of such a personal action. How much, really, could it matter?

My world was small, and I didn't concern myself with—or even consider—a big, or bigger picture.

I learned like most to stay the course, to persevere with my daily responsibilities, and to do what's right, as best I could. In short, I existed.

Of course, through crook or hook, life demands that we grow and become more than what we might want or know we need for ourselves. How else will we fulfill our own personal destinies? How else will we write our own stories? How else will we come to confront our fears, challenge our beliefs, and expand our purpose of being in the first place? How else will all those little moments growing up come to define our lives as a whole?

My personal growth began small initially…to get well.

Next, I had to find a way to rebuild my life and my business—build on what I knew, pay off my debts, and restore my credit.

Ultimately, as a result of overcoming so much adversity, and only after being forced to replace fear with tenacious defiance, did I come to my big picture—to change our health care system.

But perhaps the most profound lesson is stitched into the fabric of my world today in which only through the help of others could I have achieved so much.

There are people out there who recognize your pain and struggle, who stand ready to acknowledge your plight and are willing to help…to mentor and protect you as you make your way.

Because of the grace and gifts of others from which I benefited immensely, I strive to play it forward in all I do.

Alone, I would have accomplished little, but when joined by those who understood the challenges and were like-minded in goals, we changed the lives of many…and you can too. Standing together, you can make a difference, but someone has to be the first to stand up.

My motto today is simple: *Many voices come together when one voice stands up.*

CHAPTER 15

Forward Thinking

Today, health care is at yet, another crossroad.

Will we, as a nation, continue to pursue the private enterprise model of health care delivery while considering private/government partnerships as a means to increase both access and standards of care without sacrificing innovation?

Likewise, will the voices in favor of a more socialized or universal approach, such as Medicare for all garnish increased popularity?

What is clear is that our current system is unsustainable, from the costs involved with not only providing quality care, but expanding care to an ever-increasing population that is doomed without access.

Many believe that given my dislike of health plans, I would support a more socialized system, but they'd be wrong.

What makes our system unique is our entrepreneurial spirit, which I believe we should continue to support through private enterprise.

Regardless the systems that are put into place, history and countless studies show that prevention and personal responsibility hold the key to success.

We're eating too much of the wrong foods and expect a single-pill answer once diagnosed with diabetes, obesity, heart disease, and cancer. Regardless how we batter our bodies with fat-filled foods and processed sugar, we expect our doctors to make us better when illness strikes. We're not exercising enough, or, in the case of many, at all, expecting all the convenience of modern life without acknowledging many of the drawbacks to those conveniences. Processed foods make it possible to race through each day with little time spent planning meals, but at what costs?

The French eat sauces of cream and butter routinely, but their rate of heart disease is far less than ours because they shop for fresh, healthy foods nearby and walk almost everywhere, including the three or four flights of stairs to their apartments!

I prefer a health care system that incorporates wellness and prevention.

The "wellness and prevention" model assumes it's better for everyone to think of himself as the first line of defense against sickness.

Instead of encouraging visits to doctors, as managed care has, we should offer incentives for staying healthy. We need to follow the chronic disease/condition management program our doctors design for us and be accountable for our good health, not pawn that responsibility off on our doctor and the medical system.

We need to change our attitudes and our behavior, not to mention the example we set for our children.

Health plans also need to do their part by offering incentives and discounts for wellness and prevention. We accomplish this by education and outreach. If people do not understand their own health needs, aren't screened for possible risks, cannot obtain the healthy food choices necessary to improve their health, and cannot afford to purchase or access their medications, then how can we ever expect to change behaviors?

With incentives built into the system, we might just find our way back to better health. Those who work hard to keep themselves healthy are paying for the high costs of those who don't. Access to healthy food choices should be easily obtainable even in areas of low income and poverty. We should not have food deserts or unsafe streets.

If there's one thing that encourages consumers to act, it's saving money for them. They do not want to hear that health plans will save the money when nothing is passed on to the consumer or the employer purchasing the policies!

A great model for the management of chronic conditions/diseases is the Asheville Project, which was started by clinical pharmacists Barry Bunting and Dan Garret, members of the North Carolina Pharmacists Association, in Asheville, North Carolina, in 1997.

That the program did not receive a lot of press attention, but it doesn't take away from the fact that it is the perfect model for future wellness plans.

As a clinical hospital pharmacist, Bunting came into contact with many diseases that seemed preventable, or controllable, and in some cases, curable, especially diabetes and asthma.

Bunting, working with the North Carolina Center for Pharmaceutical Care (NCCPC) and the city of Asheville, contracted with the city to create an incentive program—first for diabetics—to work with pharmacists as their "coaches."

Originally, 1,200 city employees signed up and their pharmacist-coaches helped educate them on diet and overall diabetes prevention. It made a difference right away.

Treatment for diabetes dropped during the first year. By the fifth year, expenses for the program dropped by 40 percent, mostly because of fewer emergency room visits.

Eventually, the pilot program for diabetics expanded to asthma sufferers with equal success.

Today, plans are to steer the program toward smoking cessation and pain management and expand it to ten other cities around the country.

Regardless of how we pursue covering more of America's citizens, prevention of disease through healthier choices and lifestyles and personal accountability toward one's own health must be a driving force.

Still, there's an important role for government to play in creating national standards of coverage, including preventative services.

Today, while many tout the benefits (in terms of cost savings) of allowing individuals to purchase plans across state lines, which sounds great in theory—commonly cited for its ability to increase competition, thus reducing national premiums—there are reasons why some companies only operate out of specific states...fewer regulations.

In California, we benefit as a whole from state laws that enforce disclosure of coverage laws, continuity of care, and yes, prevention coverage, as all help to reduce the overall cost of care by ensuring a healthier population.

When an individual from another state moves to California, chances are they will arrive with health-related burdens in tow that their new employer and taxpayers will have to deal with: more costly care requirements due to lingering or out of control chronic conditions (such as heart disease or diabetes, both in many cases are preventable) that will cost more to stabilize...all due to the lack of preventative care and other health consumer assurances from back home in state they just had left.

Should someone from California suddenly be able to cross state lines and purchase health insurance from a plan based in another state, the new policy would be governed by the laws of that state, which may have fewer basic coverage mandates and consumer protections.

They may in fact experience a reduction in premium, but they'll also experience a reduction in basic coverage provided and see any savings of premium go to higher out-of-pocket expenses. Ultimately, they may forego altogether certain tests or prescription drugs recommended by their physician due to lack of coverage. Consumers who purchase out-of-state plans will be hostage to the laws (or lack of them) of the state of purchase, as California cannot enforce its laws on policies originated in another state. Of course, when such a lacking policy fails to provide for that California resident, California taxpayers will have to step up to the plate as well with increased tax dollars to fill in the blanks.

One person's exercise of free will by purchasing out-of-state health insurance would become another person's tax liability. The rhetoric today about crossing state lines to purchase insurance has caused great confusion among people in their state and added to the anxiety of uninformed consumers who listen to the media and only half of the story. Only when consumers are given the whole story can they make an informed decision, one that can make the difference between access to care and no access at all.

Without understanding each state's patient protections and coverage options consumers again will purchase a plan in the dark and not know what is covered. That same individual could surely cost California taxpayers more every year through increased emergency room visits, lack of production on the job, and ultimately, their inability to work at all due to prolonged and out of control chronic illnesses that did not have the same protections purchasing out of state had they stayed in a California-based plan.

California's insistence on basic care coverage, such as preventative care, may cost some plans revenue up front, but they make it back in spades with an overall healthier population that uses far less medical care than consumers from other states. When citizens are not forced to delay care to a point in which treatment costs are greater and outcomes more dire, the cost to taxpayers is also greatly reduced by fewer emergency room trips, less-costly procedures and less time spent off the job.

It's one thing to tout state rights, but as a nation, we sink or swim together when the health of our citizens is in jeopardy. We shouldn't forget that our federal tax dollars supplement those states that fail to protect their own as we do here in California.

Yes, there are many sides to the health care debate, and getting it right may not come anytime soon, but I'm proud that we've made enormous strides in our state and that our policies are not only proving effective at controlling costs here at home but are becoming a model for the country.

That I'm able to participate with a seat at the table in the forward thinking—inclusive and diverse discussion taking place right now—is a dream come true.

CHAPTER 16

Tomorrow Begins Today

Where does one who has been so deeply involved with patient advocacy and health care reform go from here?

Good question!

As it's clear that the twenty-first century will see enormous change, how will I best define my role and contribution to those changes? After twenty-plus years, what personal sacrifices am I willing to make to remain in the game?

Another good question!

By now my husband, Roger, was hoping that I might find a way to slow down…spend a little more time traveling with him and enjoying our friends and family, including spending a lot more time with our grandchildren.

With each challenge, I'm sure he wonders, "Will this be the one? Can she finally hang her hat on this accomplishment and leave the game on top?"

Then again, he knows me well and understands that each battle won only represents one step closer, in my mind, to the overall goal of reforming health care in a meaningful, lasting way.

To put it all in baseball terms, wouldn't that be like leaving in the ninth inning?

Ask any mother and she'll tell you that once her newborn was placed in her arms, she quickly forgot about all the toil and stress, insomnia, and discomfort that had marked her days and months leading to that eventful hour.

Each big win leaves me hungry for more because after the celebration, I'm reminded how much more needs to be done.

Still, defining what I had left in terms of "fight" or where exactly to put my efforts was difficult. For now, at least, I was happy to let gravity and the current momentum take the wheel while I fulfilled my commitments.

I've said it before, and I'll say it again: when your heart's in the right place, the way forward will be shown to you.

In late December of 2006, just as California's own health care reform debate was heating up, I received an e-mail from Governor Schwarzenegger's senior health policy director who wanted consumers to have a voice and a seat at the table. The governor was calling 2007 "The Year of Health Care Reform," and thus, a great deal needed to be accomplished as stakeholders began to negotiate in typical fashion, their perspective alliances and demands.

The idea that my dream and lifetime mission—fixing our broken health care system at the state level—was so close that I could almost reach out and touch it, and it was beyond exciting. But if I had learned anything in my years as an advocate, real reform would not come easy, quick, or without casualties.

My goal was to ensure that this time, health consumers wouldn't need to scratch and claw their way onto the field after the fact; after all the rules had been set and after their needs had been trumped in the name of profits.

No, this was an opportunity for all who had joined with me over the years to forge a strong new coalition for change.

I was asked by the CA Administration to bring together health advocate leaders for a stakeholders meeting in December of 2006 held at the Governor's office in the state capitol. I placed a call to my colleagues and together, we met just before the Christmas holiday to learn about the Administration's reform agenda and what role we saw for ourselves in the process. How could we, as health care advocates, utilize what we have learned to help foster change at in a truly meaningful way?

In all, nineteen organizations were represented at the meeting, clear about what our participation with the governor's plan could mean to their constituencies.

For me personally, it meant that I was about to embark on my most important role yet building in real time an action-oriented and engaged coalition with an agenda larger than anything we had attempted to do before.

As a loose affiliation of advocates initially, we called ourselves The Health Initiatives Working Group, where patient, provider, and social/consumer advocacy meet.

With our group's foundation woven together in strong policy development in the past, we had the power—this time—to make sweeping change in California health care. Further, we knew states across the country were looking to California to lead as well.

This was our moment, collectively...and my moment, personally.

Stepping Away from All Familiar

My work at Perry Communications had become challenging and, at times, uncomfortable. The needs of clients who might be at odds with my mission left me feeling at best, restrained, and at worst, stifled. Every move I made had some element that could be perceived, I supposed, as a conflict of interest.

Change...reform indeed, was in the air. The moment had arrived, and I wanted desperately to be free to become a part of it, but it would require personal change as well.

After expressing my thoughts and desires to Roger, who once again, stood remarkable in his support despite the impact it would have on him, I made the decision to leave my position at the public relations firm, and in doing so, I took the biggest risk of my lifetime. I wasn't sure how I was going to make a living. I just knew that I would.

From that moment on, the Working Group was all I could think about: what role would we play in challenging days ahead, where would the funding come from to build and promote our message, and how would I draw from all that I've learned to ensure that the stakeholders involved could find a way to work together?

Equally important was how, exactly, was I going to support myself in the days and months, possibly years to come?

In the near term, my mother provided the way…as always, selflessly giving to me exactly what I needed at the exactly the right time. In her recent death, my darling mom had left me a small endowment, enough to see me through as I began this new journey.

She would be so proud and pleased to know that her small endowment meant that the lives of so many would be changed and made better. I was grateful that with her help, I was allowed to seize the moment and try.

By 2007, the governor's reform plans were facing headwinds from conflicting interests and partisanship…the markers of petty disagreements that have a way of snowballing and killing progress.

As is often the case, despite the totality of incredible experience, a diverse knowledge base and decades of both successes and failures represented across the spectrum of stakeholders, the prevailing position of those charged with our future was one of protecting home plate against all odds right off the mark…or to put it another way, the notion that in order for the citizens of our state to win (true health care reform about people) surely their (representative) side would have to lose something. In a matter of no time, few could see how making health care better for people would or could support their individual gains respectfully.

Yes, the children were all seated around the table, and yet few adults among them could be found. Walls were erected and weapons of choice selected. Some had begun to simply walk away. A special meeting with the governor was called to discuss the issues that could collapse true reform. The meeting was called in a short amount of time, and again, we had a large turnout. The governor spoke as did members of his cabinet. He also listened to us, and we were not short on words.

At the time, the governor hosted a weekly Saturday morning radio show covering a wide range of issues in our state, and due to a conflict of scheduling, his administration asked me to guest host an upcoming Saturday in his absence.

Looking back, it was like having Mother Goose lay the golden egg right at my feet, but my enthusiasm for hosting the show wasn't shared amongst many in our working group.

Their fear was that by doing so, I would be aligning our group too closely to the governor's camp, which could possibly alienate some of our network supporters. But I was confident that I could make our case while also stating what we expected from all the stakeholders, the governor's office included. That was, after all, what we were known for…no special influence or treatment outside of those we were there to represent—the people—and holding everyone accountable.

Being part of a group of any kind can be challenging when the occasion arises that your personal views and ideas fall outside the majority. In our working group, no one had any more authority over another, and we always voted on agenda items and issues of concern. This time, however, because events were moving so quickly, I made a unilateral decision and moved forward without full consensus. On behalf of the group, I had been offered exclusive keys to the bully pulpit for one Saturday radio address, and it was a brass ring with an audience that I intended to grab. Luckily (for me and the working group), I was successful in delivering our collective message.

By hosting the show, I became the first and only "consumer" rather than an industry executive or government representative ever to give his (the governor's) radio address. It was an opportunity to have our coalition recognized throughout the state as a legitimate voice (on behalf of consumers) in the reform process—to let the public know we were there, fighting for them, while also challenging publicly, those stakeholders who had left the table angry, to return.

I was determined that the public have an opportunity to learn about our coalition's efforts, that we were there to fight for their right of access to quality health care, and that the reform process heed our motto: "We're about people. We're about health." We mean it!

Soon afterward, our group's working title changed to represent a more cohesive network with a clear mission, recognizing the most costly, underserved and at-risk patient group in our state—those who suffer from chronic disease. We officially became The California Chronic Care Coalition (CCCC).

(Archives: Print Version—LizHelms.Governor Schwarzenegger GuestRadioHost.10.07.PDF)

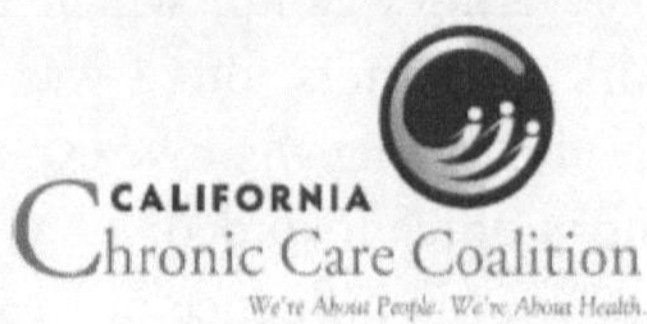

Mission Statement

- o The California Chronic Care Coalition (CCCC) is an alliance of non-profit and provider organizations united to improve the health of Californians with chronic conditions or diseases. Our mission is to improve the health care system where all Californians can access appropriate, affordable, quality health care. We do this by educating and collaborating with all branches of government and key stakeholders to re-design a system of care that includes access to appropriate affordable quality health care, including wellness and prevention coverage.

Our Vision

- o The California Chronic Care Coalition (CCCC) envisions a healthcare system where all Californians with chronic conditions or diseases can access individually appropriate health care and where people with chronic health conditions can become healthier and less costly to the healthcare system. This can be achieved through early and proper diagnosis, effective treatment, disease management, primary, secondary and tertiary prevention including timely affordable access to healthcare.

(Archive PDF)

The CCCC, with potential to have a bigger role in health care than Citizens for the Right to Know (although comprised of many of the same organizations) needed structure and organizational fortitude. The majority of 2007 was spent building that structure in both organizational framework and legal terms. It was an undertaking of massive proportions, as every detail had to be accounted for in order to begin submitting applications for grant funding, which was critical to our survival.

As chair of the CCCC, I was working from home sixteen to seventeen hours per day pulling it all together. It would be near the end of 2008 (nearly two years later) before our first grant came through from the California Endowment.

I wasn't the only one, however, working overtime without compensation to get the coalition and its goals/grants and partnerships off the ground.

While our first grant provided a much-needed financial boost to our efforts, it didn't cover everything. It didn't cover a great deal, actually.

While grants are a wonderful thing—unlike a loan, they don't need to be repaid—they are typically given for very specific items of assistance. I had included in our grant request monies to provide for one staff person who had donated to date, so much of her time to help me. The grant we received struck down that request, and even my own position as chair was only funded part-time. Had it not been for the money my mother provided me, I would not have been able to continue.

But there was much to do.

Prevention and Wellness in California: Chronic Care at Risk

The Chronic Care Coalition's number 1 goal was to stem the tide of rising costs by addressing, first and foremost, the decline of, and/or mismanaged care for those suffering from chronic conditions, as they make up the bulk of cost and represent those most at risk in any reform measure.

To that end, I had been asked to create a document outlining what the CCCC would like to see included in the governor's reform legislation moving forward as it related to chronic care specifically.

It's like yesterday in my mind. My husband, Roger, and I had taken our grandchildren to Disneyland and the question, "What do we really need?" played over and over in my head between rides, exhibits, and cotton candy crowds.

We were staying in an RV park, and one evening, as Roger and the kids turned in, exhausted from a day of Disney adventures, the answer came to me, and I began to write a roadmap of sorts—the steps necessary to prevention and wellness.

By light provided from a battery-operated lantern on a picnic table, I put pen to a pad of paper and wrote the entire Prevention and Wellness Integration Act, including legislative language in one sitting. It was as if I was the only person on the planet awake, but my mind was on fire.

The words simply flowed as if some divine entity with special access to all the files in my mind—every document of years past relating to discussions, challenges, policies, and battlegrounds—was sifting through the data and bringing the most pertinent to light in order of importance. It was as though this entity was dictating, and I was writing it all down as fast as my pen could carry the words. Once it was finished, it was sent to the coalition for their comments and edits. Not many were made, and we ended up with a document that has been used by many ever since.

Ultimately, the document was voted on and approved for inclusion, and our first victory took place when the Assembly passed the governor's health care reform bill. All stakeholders came to the press conference that followed the vote. Business, health plans, unions, consumers, advocates, providers, and physicians all attend. It was an amazing high-energy day. We were so sure the bill would pass the Senate and become the model law for the country (we had worked out many of the issues Massachusetts and learned from them what to correct.)

However, the governor's health reform bill was voted down in the senate—a *political* move that was devastating after all the hard work done by so many to help it pass. Our coalition worked tireless on the bill and poured its heart and soul into the effort nonstop. It was as if we experienced a blowout on the freeway so close to our destination and crashed without warning.

The governor called a press conference that was, despite the circumstances, uplifting, ensuring that we would not give up, not stop our drive for reform.

All was not lost. Not only did key features of the act I wrote find their way into California's own health reform language, the Prevention and Wellness Act ultimately made its way to Washington where a great deal of its language was included in the Affordable Care Act itself as must-have preventative care benefits to be included in the exchanges that would take effect at the state level in 2014.

Could I be more proud of our efforts?

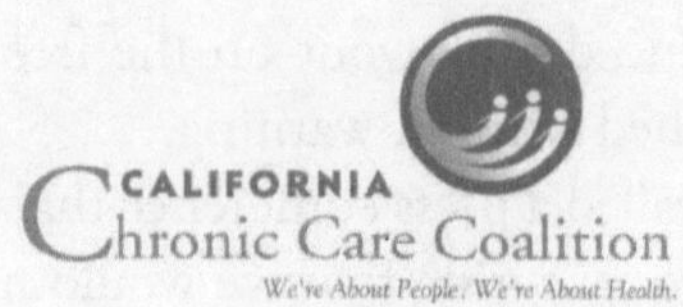

July 17, 2008
Prevention and Wellness Integration Act for the Management of Chronic Conditions

The Legislature finds and declares that:

1. Best practices for care of people with 'chronic conditions should serve as a starting point for the restructuring of health care delivery.' (Institutes of Medicine)

2. Chronic conditions/diseases are the primary driver of health care costs accounting for more than 75 cents of every dollar being spent on health care, as reported by the Centers for Disease Control (CDC).

3. Many Californians with a chronic condition have more than one chronic condition (co-morbidities). Co-morbidities not only create a greater risk of disability, but they complicate treatment and create a greater risk of hospitalization or institutionalization.

4. Affordable patient-centered care that provides access to all three levels of prevention, (primary, secondary and tertiary), is cost-effective over the course of the disease or condition. It will reduce or eliminate unnecessary hospitalizations, surgery, physician visits, and nursing home admissions.

5. Patient-centered access to prevention should include the utilization of multi-disciplinary teams for development, management of treatment and care.

6. People with chronic conditions have complex needs, which California's healthcare delivery system must address. With hospital costs accounting for the bulk of healthcare spending in California, one goal of health reform must be to improve management of chronic conditions and diseases and reducing hospitalizations.

7. Assessing the family caregiver and developing a plan for their support and education in caring for the family member's care needs will improve outcomes, lowering hospitalizations and other institutional care.

909 12th Street. Suite 201. Sacramento, CA 95814
916 444-1985 office ◆ 916 300-8687 direct
www.chroniccareca.org

8. Promoting wellness, chronic disease prevention, educating patients and improving access for all Californians to patient-centered, primary care medical homes, throughout the private and public health care system, will improve the health of Californians.

9. Promoting healthy lifestyles in workplaces, schools and communities by collaborating with business, faith-based, not-for-profit health organizations, education, including school health centers, government and other community leaders, can lead to sustainable changes in health behaviors.

10. Improving the quality and availability of health information technology (HIT) throughout the health care system, data collection and consumer access to their personal medical records, will improve overall care management.

11. Medication therapy management is readily available to patients with chronic conditions and diseases, where the pharmacist is working collaboratively with the treating physician(s), and provides individualized care. This will reduce the risk of adverse events, including adverse drug interactions, improve compliance and will better manage chronic conditions.

RESOLVED: That the California Legislature add Section XXXX to the Health and Safety Code to read as follows:
Section ___________

The Department of Public Health, the Department of Health and Human Services and the Department of Insurance shall establish and maintain the Prevention and Wellness Integration Act of 2008 for the management of chronic conditions, including, but not limited to the following:

1. Restructuring health care systems to:
   (a) Include in all benefit plan designs coverage for primary and preventive care services, including prescription drugs, combined with all levels that promote prevention for management of chronic conditions.
   (b) Develop, with assistance of public/private and community partnerships, the promotion of wellness and chronic disease prevention, utilizing early intervention tools and management models incorporated throughout private and public health care systems.
   (c) Promote a culture of health care productivity through the use of multi-disciplinary, primary care medical home models, medication therapy management, and patient-centered access to all three levels of prevention (primary, secondary, tertiary).
   (d) Promotion of healthy lifestyles in workplaces, schools and communities by establishing a collaborative between business, health plans, faith-based, not-for-profit health organizations, consumer groups, education, including school health

The Affordable Care Act and the California Exchange

The year 2009 became for the nation what 2007 was to California on steroids—the year of health care reform at the national level, which is to say, an explosive public discourse that would once again pit stakeholders against each other and the country as special interests maneuvered to secure their positions, at risk once again of forgetting the most important reason for reform, patients and their needs… their right to access quality and affordable health care.

I watched with both fascination and grave concern as the country stood at the precipitous of what many before Obama had tried to achieve: health care reform that could stem the tide of rising costs, while also providing for those who found access difficult, if not impossible, as well as those who, in spite of coverage, were under-insured or dropped from their coverage when diagnosed with a chronic or acute illness.

Since the Affordable Care Act's passage in 2010, many states chose to forestall vital planning and implementation efforts in lieu of expected and impending court challenges to the act itself. Of course, we now know that the U.S. Supreme Court has upheld the ACA, thus forcing states to comply by either organizing an exchange, or having one created for them by the feds.

In 2010, the mission of the California Chronic Care Coalition, however, was to move the ball forward in our state, regardless how things were playing out in Washington.

California, committed to health care reform regardless the outcome at the national level, pushed onward with two important pieces of legislation immediately.

One, the establishment of a state-managed exchange to provide cost-effective health plans as outlined in the Affordable Care Act, beginning in 2014.

Secondly, to provide coverage for individuals with preexisting conditions as a stop-gap measure…a means to provide temporary health insurance until such time (2014) that all health plans are mandated to accept individuals with preexisting conditions.

The state legislature had before it, a bill to begin the implementation of a state health insurance exchange. As Washington heated up over the Affordable Care Act, Republicans in our state were hard-pressed to enact legislation that could be seen as an extension of or helpful to what was coming to be known as "Obama Care."

While mandatory state exchanges—as part of the Affordable Care Act—wouldn't go into effect until 2014, a great deal needed to happen long before then in order to provide for the millions who would suddenly become eligible for coverage. New health care facilities throughout the state need to be built, along with an effective means of hiring new physicians and support staff, such as RNs, LVNs, PAs, clinical pharmacists, clinicians, and technicians. For their part, the federal government was offering grant funds to ensure that states had the resources to begin such an undertaking.

But the states are also charged with how those exchanges will function based on the ACA—the basics of coverage, levels of individual participation, and support for small and large businesses that offer health coverage to their employees.

To move forward, the California Exchange bill had to be passed.

As the vote neared and it was clear the measure was in danger of failing due to political pressure, the CCCC met with legislators to educate them and brought with them factual state data. We pushed the stakeholders of our coalition to the max, everyone on deck making the case for patients over politics…for the people of our state, as they were the ultimate stakeholders who were counting on us and the legislators to do our jobs. For me, I went to every legislator in the building passing out letters and letting them know the CCCC supported a CA Exchange.

The day of the vote, many of our groups along with the California Medical Association formed a team and met with a key legislator we knew was still undecided. We discussed the reasons why we believed CA needed to take the lead and protect our consumers rather than the feds making the rules. If CA decided to have its own Health Benefits Exchange, we would still be able to make decisions on how to set it up by using federal guidelines still keeping California's vast and diverse populations under the scrutiny of our state. This way, stakeholders would have a voice in the decision-making process and people that know our state best would be setting the rules.

And it worked. One hour after, our meeting finished, and holding our breath, the vote was taken. The legislator we met with listened to our voices and voted in favor of the exchange. That was the one voted needed to turn the tide and pass the bill. It was an amazing moment, one that held both the promise of a new dawn in California health care, as well as a shot of "well done" for the coalition. We were on our way to transforming care, making a real and substantial difference. Even more so, we had earned our stripes as a force to be acknowledged and respected proving that those with different agendas and goals can indeed come together at the same table and work hard to overcome our differences. At some point, Californians will realize having our own state-based Health Benefits Exchange was in the best interest for everyone. Again our work had only just begun, and we needed to be sure the exchange was developed to improve access to quality health care with a focus on prevention, wellness, and better management of chronic conditions/diseases.

Now on to basic benefit design…

California Patient Protection and Affordability Care Act—*California Exchange*

```
BILL NUMBER: AB 1602      CHAPTERED
      BILL TEXT

      CHAPTER  655
      FILED WITH SECRETARY OF STATE   SEPTEMBER 30, 2010
      APPROVED BY GOVERNOR   SEPTEMBER 30, 2010
      PASSED THE SENATE   AUGUST 24, 2010
      PASSED THE ASSEMBLY   AUGUST 25, 2010
      AMENDED IN SENATE   AUGUST 20, 2010
      AMENDED IN SENATE   AUGUST 17, 2010
      AMENDED IN SENATE   AUGUST 2, 2010
      AMENDED IN SENATE   JUNE 24, 2010
      AMENDED IN ASSEMBLY   APRIL 15, 2010
      AMENDED IN ASSEMBLY   APRIL 8, 2010

INTRODUCED BY   Assembly Member John A. Perez
   (Principal coauthors: Assembly Members Bass and Monning)
   (Principal coauthors: Senators Alquist and Steinberg)

                  JANUARY 5, 2010

   An act to amend Sections 15438 and 15439 of, and to add Sections
100501, 100502, 100503, 100504, 100505, 100506, 100507, 100508,
100520, and 100521 to, the Government Code, to add Section 1366.6 to
the Health and Safety Code, and to add Section 10112.3 to the
Insurance Code, relating to health care coverage, and making an
appropriation therefor.
```

California Patient Protection and Affordability Care Act—*California Exchange*

Continued

THE PEOPLE OF THE STATE OF CALIFORNIA DO ENACT AS FOLLOWS:

SECTION 1. This act shall be known and may be cited as the California Patient Protection and Affordable Care Act.

SEC. 2. It is the intent of the Legislature to enact the necessary statutory changes to California law in order to establish an American Health Benefit Exchange in California and its administrative authority in a manner that is consistent with the federal Patient Protection and Affordable Care Act (Public Law 111-148), as amended by the federal Health Care and Education Reconciliation Act of 2010 (Public Law 111-152), hereafter the federal act. In doing so, it is the intent of the Legislature to do all of the following:

(a) Reduce the number of uninsured Californians by creating an organized, transparent marketplace for Californians to purchase affordable, quality health care coverage, to claim available federal tax credits and cost-sharing subsidies, and to meet the personal responsibility requirements imposed under the federal act.

(b) Strengthen the health care delivery system.

(c) Guarantee the availability and renewability of health care coverage through the private health insurance market to qualified individuals and qualified small employers.

(d) Require that health care service plans and health insurers issuing coverage in the individual and small employer markets compete on the basis of price, quality, and service, and not on risk selection.

(e) Meet the requirements of the federal act and all applicable federal guidance and regulations.

http://www.leginfo.ca.gov/pub/09-10/bill/asm/ab_1601-1650/ab_1602_bill_20100930_chaptered.html

Pre-Existing Conditions: Denied and Discouraged

As stated at www.chronicaareca.org, in 2005, 133 million Americans—almost one out of every two adults—had at least one chronic illness, what is considered to be a preexisting condition when applying for health care coverage.

As part of the Affordable Care Act, California residents who are unable to secure health insurance due to a preexisting condition are now able to apply for the California Pre-Existing Condition Insurance Plan (PCIP), a federally funded stopgap program established to help provide for high-risk consumers.

The program is available until December 13, 2013, when all insurance plans nationally will be required to cover persons with pre-existing conditions without discrimination or higher rates.

As the CCCC's heart and soul is devoted to the improved care for those suffering chronic and acute health conditions, I applaud California's efforts to both inform residents about available coverage through PCIP and their tireless work to improve the program in ways that enhance care while striving to reduce unwarranted costs.

For a complete overview of the program, including how to apply, visit: http://www.pcip.ca.gov/Home/default.aspx

But I digress. Back to the Chronic Care Coalition and our future, together.

While the national discussion regarding health care reform raged, the CCCC had been hard at work at home with partners throughout our state, advancing cutting-edge programs with achievable wellness goals in our sights.

The Right Care Initiative Project

In all my travels and participation in various collaborative efforts, initiatives, and coalitions, while policy was at the forefront, integration at the street level—where policy interacts with the patients and works—is the pot at the end of the rainbow for me.

Finally, a chance to put into practice what I and the CCCC had been preaching became a reality.

In March of 2008, the Department of Managed Care, the University of California Los Angeles, UC Berkeley Schools of Public Health, and the RAND Corporation joined in partnership with an expert-based, private/public, multi-year collaborative called the Right Care Initiative (RCI). The initiative launch of the RCI was in 2008. The California Chronic Care Coalition joined RCI in 2009.

Such a collaborative is exactly the kind that the strengths and experience of the CCCC came to be known for, and quite frankly, it represented our favorite type of playground because it was at the 'people' level, where what you do and who you help can be seen in real time. We quickly got to work and rolled up our sleeves.

The initiative's goals were to apply scientific evidence and out-come improvement strategies for the purpose of reducing deaths, while at the same time, increasing the quality of health within California's 15 million managed health plan member groups.

In English, that means we were about to take the best of what really works, mix it with tools on the cutting edge of health care, and put it into action on the streets within a community to see how much of a difference we could make.

Right Care centered its early objectives on three targeted areas:

- hypertension and cardiovascular disease
- diabetes
- hospital acquired infections

In essence, Right Care was about providing a community-fo-cused education and wellness effort utilizing care providers within the medical groups and clinics, retail pharmacy outlets, and clini-cal pharmacy directors to achieve improved blood pressure, lipids, and glucose levels—within the 90 percent nationally—thus reduc-ing disability and death due to strokes, heart attacks, and diabetic complications.

The goals were aggressive, targeted, and well supported.

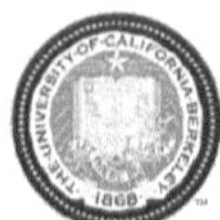 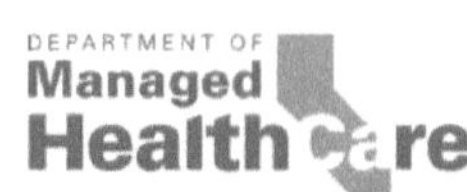 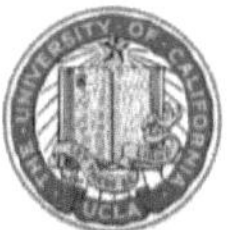

RIGHT CARE INITIATIVE *Clinical Quality Improvement Leadership Collaborative*

California Statewide Goals—Preventing Heart Attacks, Strokes, and Diabetic Complications

Achieve National HEDIS 90th Percentile "A-grade" Targets (2013 Performance Year):
 75% of hypertensive patients with **blood pressure controlled:** <140/90 mm Hg
 70% of patients with cardiovascular conditions with **lipids properly managed** (proxy: controlled to LDL-C < 100 mg/dL)
 69% of diabetic patients with **blood sugar controlled:** HbA1c <8
 56% of diabetic patients with **lipids controlled:** LDL-C < 100 mg/dL
 55% of diabetic patients with **blood pressure controlled:** <140/80 mm Hg

Current Activities:
- **University of Best Practices** in three metropolitan areas to share learning and encourage adoption of evidence-based interventions for preventing heart attacks, strokes, and complications from diabetes (e.g., amputations, blindness, kidney failure). Practical presentations from benchmark performers are geared toward medical, pharmacy and quality improvement directors, coupled with free Continuing Medical Education in Sacramento and Los Angeles, to spur achievement of national "A-grade" performance.
- **Annual leadership summit** to highlight newly released HEDIS & P4P performance data, award top performers and QI leaders, and promote adoption of strategies used by leading edge *Triple Aim* performers. 8th Annual Summit 11-5-15.

Contact: Hattie Rees Hanley, MPP, Right Care Initiative Director, hattie.hanley@dmhc.ca.gov; hattiehanley@berkeley.edu

Key Partners: This collaborative, expert-based, public-private bridge project draws on leadership from key partners:

.CA Dept. of Managed Health Care	.Sierra Health Foundation	.American Heart/Stroke Association
.CA medical groups, clinics & health plans	.American Medical Group Assoc.	.California Endowment
.University of California schools of public health, pharmacy, and medicine	.CA Office of the Patient Advocate	.California Health Care Foundation
	.CA Medi-Cal Program (DHCS)	.Ralphs Grocery Company
.Stanford Clinical Excellence Research Center	.CA Dept. of Public Health (CDPH)	.Novo Nordisk
.University of Southern California	.Integrated Healthcare Assoc. (IHA)	.Genentech
.California Chronic Care Coalition	.Pacific Business Group on Health	.Boehringer-Ingelheim
.Health Services Advisory Group QIO	.US Department of Veteran's Affairs	.Johnson & Johnson .Abbvie

Objective: Measurably reduce death and disability through enhanced practice of patient-centered, evidence-based medicine. Since 2007, The Right Care Initiative's goal has been to apply scientific evidence and outcomes improvement strategies to reduce patient morbidity and mortality through a collaborative focus on achieving quality goals where performance metrics indicate that evidence-based, life-saving practices are not fully deployed. Data from the Integrated Health Care Association, the National Committee For Quality Assurance, the federal Agency for Health Care Quality and Research, the Commonwealth Foundation, CMS, and the Centers for Disease Control indicate that approximately 81,000 Californians die yearly from heart attacks, strokes and diabetic complications. Many of these deaths and associated disabilities and health care costs could be prevented with evidence-based patient management and clinical quality improvement to adopt up to date medical knowledge. Our work is focused in these high-leverage areas of better management of **cardiovascular disease and diabetes, with** particular emphasis on **control of blood pressure, cholesterol and blood sugar.**

CDPH estimates Californians suffer approximately **72,000 deaths from cardiovascular disease** (including heart attack and stroke) and **7,000 deaths from diabetes each year**, many of them preventable according to CDC. NCQA conservatively estimates that improving California's cardiovascular disease and diabetes measures to the national HEDIS 90th percentile could save 1,694 to 2,818 CA lives each year, while avoiding $118 million in yearly hospital costs, 766,401 sick days and $125.56 million in lost productivity. Heart disease, hypertension and diabetes are increasingly well understood scientifically, and ripe for best practices collaboration. Over the course of this project, California has outpaced the nation in improving health system performance on control of blood pressure, cholesterol and blood sugar, building on the "100,000 Lives" campaign for reducing medical errors and the Million Hearts™ national initiative launched in 2011.

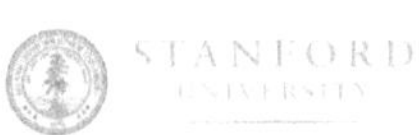 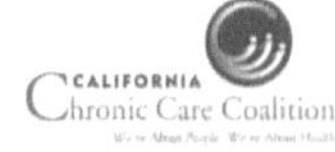

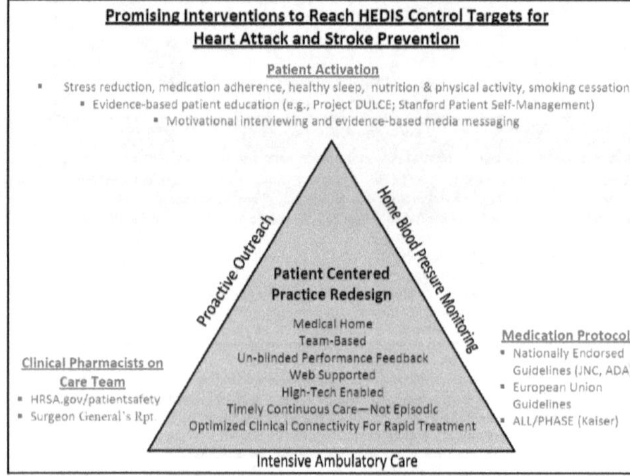

San Diego University of Best Practices steering committee medical directors came to consensus that *heart attacks and strokes could be reduced by 50% in 5 years by implementing the interventions on the Right Care Triangle*.

Research Questions:

- What are the promising interventions for bringing patients into safe control?

- How can implementation of evidence-based medicine be refined to quickly meet the Right Care goals and what are the barriers for doing so?

- What strategies are needed to improve clinical outcomes in light of health disparities in California's diverse population?

Be There San Diego: Patient Activation and Engagement in Motion

Right Care represented for me what I had longed for from the beginning: an opportunity to prove that it was possible to improve care, improve outcomes for patients, and at the same time, prove that you could reduce the costs of health care if everyone came together in common cause.

Through the Right Care Initiative, I was embarking on the most important journey yet, able to actually change health care through advocacy in action by drawing on all I had learned and those whom I had built relationships with along the way.

Thanks to a grant by the National Institute of Health, the Right Care Initiative was able to choose its first community in which to pilot the program, and the CCCC would play a leading organizational role in its implementation.

Based upon its diverse and consolidated population, as well as the limited number of health plans serving the area, San Diego was selected to become the pilot of what would eventually, if successful, expand to a statewide program.

The challenges were great, but the rewards would be immeasurable if we could pull it off.

It didn't take long before it was obvious that I would need to be on the ground in San Diego more than I had originally anticipated, and growing weary of hotel rooms, I gave in and rented a small apartment. Roger held down the fort in Sacramento, and I flew home as much as possible.

Be There® San Diego catalyzed by the Right Care Initiative platform setting up audacious goals that could only be successful by engaging primary care providers and specialists, hospitals and neighborhood clinics, corner pharmacies and large chains alike, and the community at large with a significant educational campaign.

With the help and support of the San Diego Chargers former kicker, Rolf Benirschke, (a true patient advocate himself) and a "who's who" list of some of the country's most leading medical researchers, facilities, and advanced technologies located in southern California, individuals and communities were encouraged to participate, to take charge of their health, to get the information they needed to support a healthy lifestyle, and to take pride in what their community, as a whole, could achieve in reduced heart attacks and strokes.

The message was a simple one: When you care for your own health, you're able to "be there" for those you love.

Easy-to-use, innovative, and advanced technologies, such as wireless heart monitors and smart phones with unique software for tracking your success, were to be made available to participants.

Health screening events and our multimedia campaign was defined!

And most importantly, vital integration of San Diego County's health community was established, everyone working together to get people the *right* care and education at the *right* time.

There it was…My dream was coming true.

The CCCC's Ongoing Role in Chronic Care and the Affordable Care Act

In January (2012), as we continued to advocate for patients both in San Diego and throughout the state, the CCCC participated in a vital discussion regarding the Affordable Care Act and what the new law outlined as Essential Health Benefits (EHB).

A primary goal of the ACA is to ensure that all health plans, including the exchanges created by individual states, offer a basic, comprehensive package of services known as "essential health benefits" (EHB) spanning ten categories, including, but not limited to emergency services, hospitalization, maternity and newborn care, mental health, prescription drugs, and pediatric services.

Also included in the EHB guideline is preventative and wellness services and chronic disease management.

When offered the opportunity to comment and submit recommendations, the CCCC provided the U.S. Health and Human Services department with a proposal based upon the many hard-earned advancements in preventative care that California residents now enjoy.

Recognizing that the manner in which the federal government designs and employs the EHB will greatly impact consumers, and potentially, could erode current California law, the CCCC encouraged the EHB to follow the California Knox-Keene Act, which ensures important protections for patients, providers and plans themselves.

Think of where we are now in health care reform as the big leagues. It's no longer just about California, but the nation as a whole, and fortunately, the CCCC's role in both state and federal legislation continues to keep the needs of patients—health care consumers—at the heart of the discussion.

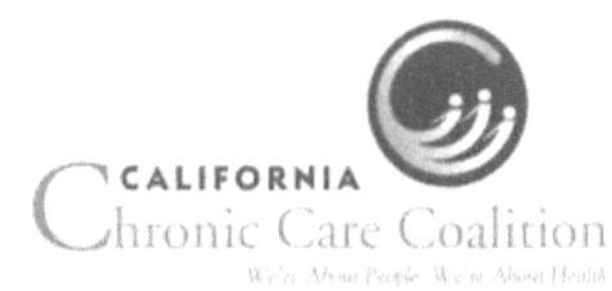

Essential Health Benefits (EHB)
US Health and Human Services

January 31, 2012

California Chronic Care Coalition Comments

Thank you for giving the California Chronic Care Coalition (CCCC) the opportunity to provide comments on the Essential Benefits. **The California Chronic Care Coalition** (CCCC) is an alliance of non-profit and provider organizations united to improve the health of Californians. Our mission is to improve the health care system so that all Californians with chronic conditions can access appropriate quality health care. CCCC encourages prevention, including effective diagnosis and management of chronic disease within California healthcare policies.

The way in which the federal government designs the "Essential Benefits" will directly impact California patient access to quality care, and the lives of millions of Californians, including those living with chronic disease, will depend on whether Essential Benefits are inclusive, affordable and meet patient needs.

> *The California Chronic Care Coalition proposes the following recommendations to focus on the alarming growth of chronic conditions and a road map to better manage complex chronic diseases through comprehensive coverage. Access to affordable, adequate coverage that enables health care access is critically important for people with, and at risk for, complex chronic diseases/conditions. When people are not able to afford the tools and care necessary to manage their chronic conditions, they scale back or forego the care they need, which often leads to complications and suffering that could have been prevented. That means an expensive trip to the emergency room and hospital readmissions that could have been avoided.*

A Journey Continues: Pride and Gratitude

For the last several years, I've divided my life and advocacy efforts between Sacramento and San Diego, traveling back and forth as both the coordinator of "Be There" San Diego campaign and my ongoing role as president/CEO of the CCCC as we continue our work on behalf of California health care consumers statewide through legislative and other partnership means.

Roger would love nothing more than for me to join him in retirement so that together, we could enjoy our favorite pastime, traveling. He would prefer that I collaborate on the most important issue of all…us. And there's a part of me that would like nothing better than the open road, my Roger at the helm of our travel RV, and of course, my horse trailer in tow. Destination…anywhere USA.

But here's the rub: I'm there, finally achieving my dream, finally making a difference that I can see in tangible terms…a real and substantial difference in the lives of health care consumers, both within our state and potentially, nationally.

The numbers out of San Diego prove it.

Still, statewide and nationally, we are at a critical stage—a crossroads of sort in which the decisions we make now will affect us for decades to come. Can I really stop now?

For all the years, I've been involved with health care advocacy, my goal, and that of the amazing organizations I've been honored to work with has been to pursue policy that was based on people—the right care at the right time.

Today, as stakeholders come together, be they representative of private or government entities, factors of population, and metric-based health care, and quality of life are at the center of the discussion.

Regardless the stakeholder, I hear over and over familiar questions: If one's quality of life can no longer be sustained or returned to a previous healthy state, where do we draw the line in care received? At what point is "extension" of life without "quality" of life a factor in denial of care?

What they're really saying is, "If we draw the line at providing care up to and including a goal of say, 50 percent—quality of life—recovery, what happens to those who are at, perhaps 49 percent or 45 percent with assistance?"

And the discussion is still based, first and foremost, on cost, not people.

I cannot accept this.

I believed initially, and do so still today, that when the right treatment is given to the right patient at the right time—treatment, as deemed necessary and appropriate by a physician in conjunction with the desires of his/her patient—cost savings can be found in science-based medicine that considers the individual.

Decades may have passed from when I first entered this debate, but this truth is no less so today. And yet here we are…again.

With Each New Perspective

Health care science in the United States is on the brink of incredible discovery.

Today, a patient is able to stand in a room and have the walls light up with 3-D images of their entire body—one multi-screen MRI, if you will, where physicians can see the total body involvement of disease or injury.

Innovative scientific advancement includes preventative care based on known DNA principals—your unique code that determines what, if any, cancers are you prone to, what metabolic tendencies are dictating your susceptibility to diabetes, and what specific medications will best address your medical condition while avoiding unnecessary complications and/or negative reactions…all based upon your unique DNA.

It's already here, and the technology would blow your mind.

And more importantly, as we stand on the cusp of such amazing medical achievements, who exactly will determine when, where, and for whom these advancements in care will be offered?

I believe with all my heart that I was born for the role I am playing today. My personal struggles with TMD and my role as founder of The TMJ Society gave me exposure to a world once foreign, and quite literally, against me.

Being a member of Citizens for the Right to Know, and of course, the invaluable experience I gained in public relations with Perry Communications Group have all been foundational…stepping stones to where I am today, which would have been impossible otherwise.

The many committed patient advocacy organizations and the leaders within them have taught me so much about caring for the "whole" of people.

As "Be There" San Diego enjoys incredible success, soon to be on autopilot as the B initiative Be-There Patient/Provider Activation and public awareness campaign expands to other communities throughout the state, I have returned to Sacramento full time.

As for retirement, I have no doubt that I'll know when it's time: when that moment appears like a soft whisper from my heart that I've accomplished all that I set out to do, and that it's time to pass the reins on to another equally capable.

But until then, I remain unwavering in my commitment, always with purpose, and ever striving to ensure that California continues to lead the nation in health care reform—that the health and well-being of our consumers is central, rather than an afterthought in the discussion.

It's my most sincere hope that you've been inspired by my story and encouraged to follow your own purposeful yearnings…to be a participant in life rather than on the sidelines, and as my dear friend Renee Paper stated, "You either play the deck you are handed or fold. I am playing."

I hope you'll take a moment to review the resources and ongoing programs outlined at our website: www.healthcareunhinged.com.

My ultimate success will be determined by the success of others who continue to play it forward, so please, join a health care coalition or community health initiative helping others in your area. There's a place for everyone…a seat at every table if only you stand as one voice among many, speaking out together.

Meanwhile, stay tuned for there is more, much more to come!

To learn more about the many ways you can become involved, as well as the Right Care Initiative or any of the programs supported by the California Chronic Care Coalition, visit us online at http://www.chroniccareca.org.

To the future, and your continued good health!

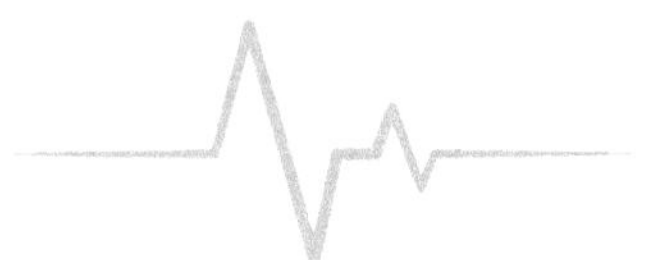

ABOUT THE AUTHOR

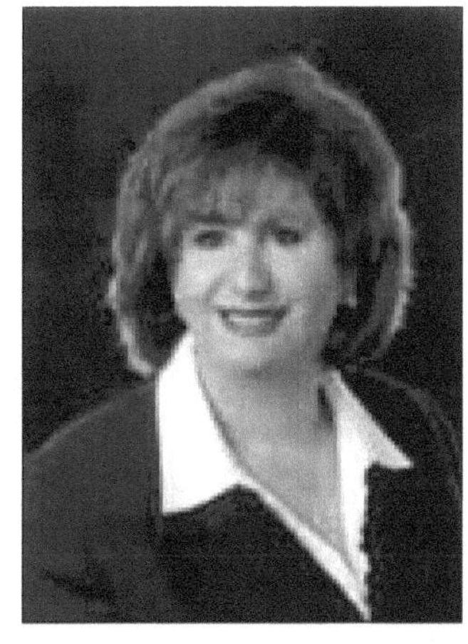

In 1993, Liz Helms learned what it meant to be invisible within a profitable California healthcare system that failed to acknowledge the needs of many, and worse, a changing industry that had until then, operated with near impunity. That was then ...before the once small business shop-owner-turned-advocate decided that the old rules were insufficient to manage the state's growing health consumer population and their challenges.

If she and the state's then 32 million others were to survive the transformation of private insurance to a system dominated by HMO and PPO care plans, consumers were going to have to be better educated, standards of care would need the protections afforded by state law, and the insurance industry itself would have to become more responsive and transparent.

In 1995, Liz founded the non-profit (501c), TMJ Society of California, an advocacy organization to advance the treatment of, and right to insurance coverage for those who, like herself, had suffered a traumatic muscular-facial jaw injury, and spearheaded a movement that resulted in passage of AB 2994, the Jaw Joint Bill.

Having been educated early on to the disparities suffered by so many with chronic or acute illnesses, Liz lead a kitchen-table coalition of committed professionals into a statewide coalition of some 80 stakeholders to support a citizen's *'Right to Know'*.

Representing tens of thousands of California residents who found themselves lost in a system lacking access to quality care and complicated, if not hidden policy agendas, Liz has told her story and that of others on the floor of the California state legislature during numerous hearings over the years, as well as before congress of the United States and the National Institutes of Health, each time breaking through barriers of indifference to put a face on those often left behind in their considerations and deliberations of law.

Over the course of twenty years, the name Liz Helms has become synonymous with coalition building, grassroots advocacy, strategic planning and progressive policy development, capable of bridging relationships that had in the past, maintained a distant, if not oppositional status.

On behalf of California consumers, in 2006, she forged new ground as the co-founder and President of the California Chronic Care Coalition, contributing valuable policy insight for California health reform in 2007 and during the drafting of the ACA, uniting the chronic disease community throughout the state.

Through Liz's stewardship of the heralded *Right Care Initiative*, San Diego became the first California community to begin working toward achieving a heart attack and stroke-free zone. She continues to expand the outreach and partnership efforts of the Chronic Care Coalition throughout northern California inspiring multi-front cardiovascular care initiatives within underserved communities, and played a pivotal in a vital 2015 ruling by Covered California to limit individual out-of-pocket costs for acute, chronic care patients in need of expensive, life-saving drugs that had been classified outside of standard drug formularies by insurance companies.

Her work on behalf of patients' rights and advocacy has helped millions